HEALING
Gourmet®
Eat to Lower
Cholesterol

HEALING
Gourmet®
Eat to Lower Cholesterol

THE EDITORS OF HEALING GOURMET WITH

Victoria Rand, M.D.,

Kathy McManus, M.S., RD, and Bev Shaffer

McGraw-Hill

New York   Chicago   San Francisco   Lisbon   London   Madrid   Mexico City
Milan   New Delhi   San Juan   Seoul   Singapore   Sydney   Toronto

The McGraw·Hill Companies

Library of Congress Cataloging-in-Publication Data

Healing gourmet eat to lower cholesterol / with Victoria Rand, Kathy McManus, and Bev Shaffer.
  p.   cm.
Includes bibliographical references and index.
ISBN 0-07-146198-1 (alk. paper)
  1. Low-cholesterol diet—Popular works.   2. Low-cholesterol diet—Recipes.
I. McManus, Kathy.   II. Shaffer, Bev, 1951–.   III. Title.

RM237.75.R36   2005
641.5'6311—dc22   2005017028

2 3 4 5 6 7 8 9 0   FGR/FGR   0 9 8 7 6

ISBN 0-07-146198-1

Interior design by Monica Baziuk

McGraw-Hill books are available at special quantity discounts to use as premiums and sales promotions, or for use in corporate training programs. For more information, please write to the Director of Special Sales, Professional Publishing, McGraw-Hill, Two Penn Plaza, New York, NY 10121-2298. Or contact your local bookstore.

This book is printed on acid-free paper.

This book is dedicated to those with high cholesterol or living with heart disease.

Contents

Acknowledgments

THIS BOOK IS brought to you with the assistance and knowledge of medical, culinary, and nutrition experts from across the nation, as well as the diligent work of countless scientists worldwide who help us to translate "research to recipes" in our mission to educate on the link between diet and disease. Healing Gourmet would like to thank the following people for their contributions.

A very special thanks to our book editor Natasha Graf for her attention to detail and function as catalyst for many of the concepts presented in the book, and to our project editor, Nancy Hall, for her excellent work in the final editing of the manuscript.

Our medical, nutrition, and culinary editors: thanks to Dr. Victoria Rand for her thorough review and guidance; to Kathy McManus for her speedy and meticulous work on recipe analysis, meal planning, and nutritional review; and Bev Shaffer for her culinary expertise to ensure our recipes deliver as much taste as they do health. A special thanks to Chef Paul Jones for running the Healing Gourmet test kitchen.

Our publisher: thanks to McGraw-Hill for their commitment to delivering high-quality information to the public, including many of the educational textbooks that spurred the development of this company.

Our affiliations: thanks to the fine institutions that bring us these editors including Harvard Medical School, Brigham and Women's Hospital, University of California at San Francisco, and the Cleveland Clinic Foundation.

Our associates and family: thanks to Guy Gelin and our friends and families for their continuing support of the Healing Gourmet project.

Introduction

HEALING GOURMET BEGAN with a mission to educate people on the link between diet and disease. As part of a series, this book is meant to provide useful information on eating to beat high cholesterol through sound nutritional principles. We bring the "clinic" together with the "kitchen" to help you deliciously make the most of your health through the latest discoveries. Quite simply, Healing Gourmet translates "research to recipes," making your kitchen a healing haven.

In this book, we will help you to understand the basic principles of cholesterol and how your diet can help to manage your condition and prevent complications. Chapters 1 and 2 focus on how cholesterol affects heart disease, what the numbers mean, the factors that contribute to your cholesterol levels, and the lifestyle changes to help you take control. In Chapters 3 and 4, we'll give you the skinny on fat and the truth about carbohydrates; we'll introduce you to your cholesterol-lowering arsenal of phytonutrients and antioxidants. In Chapters 5 and 6, we give you the delicious foods and the herbs and spices where you can find these nutrients.

Of course, we'll help you to sleuth out the healthiest products at the grocery in Chapter 7, plan your heart-healthy meals in Chapter 8, and give you fifty great recipes to get started in

Chapter 9. Don't forget to visit our website, healinggourmet.com, for the latest research and more heart-healthy recipes!

Important disclaimer: the information in this book cannot replace the advice of your physician or health-care team. Always consult with your doctor or dietitian before making any changes in diet.

Letter from the Editor

CAN SOMETHING AS delicious as a Mediterranean Baked Snapper help to lower your cholesterol and stifle heart disease? This is just one of the questions we set out to answer nearly five years ago with the creation of our company. Dedicated solely to helping the public make better choices about the foods to eat to prevent disease, Healing Gourmet brings you sound, scientific evidence and practical solutions to help you take control of your health.

Our recipe for health is simple. First, we take a disease-fighting dose of research collected from the National Library of Medicine on your favorite foods, compounds in foods, and their effects on disease. Right at this very moment, scientists are hard at work analyzing nutrients in foods for their beneficial effects on blood sugar, their cholesterol-lowering capacity, and their cholesterol-lowering action. Other researchers are poring over data from population studies to give us clues to why disease rates are lower in other countries where the diets differ greatly from those in the United States. Together, this research in the "new nutritional frontier" acts as the foundation—the first ingredient—in a cholesterol-lowering mix. To help us in this research, we are extremely fortunate to have the assistance of Victoria Rand, M.D. Dr. Rand is an assistant clinical professor of medicine in the Department of Medicine at the University of California at San Francisco and is board certified in internal medicine with training in acupuncture, herbal medicine, and other complementary therapies. The next step in our recipe for health is incorporating these scientific findings with culinary finesse to whip up mouthwatering recipes and easy-to-use meal plans that help you make the most of the latest nutritional breakthroughs. For this task, we are also lucky to have the expertise and nutritional analysis of Kathy McManus, M.S., RD—the director of nutrition at Brigham and Women's Hospital—and the culinary expertise of Chef Bev Shaffer, culinary director of the "Cooking with Your Heart" Program in association with the Cleveland Clinic Foundation.

Don't forget to visit us on the Web at healinggourmet.com and look for us on television this fall debuting on the Healthy Living Channel. Enjoy these books in good health and *eat your medicine*!

—KELLEY LUNSFORD
Editor-in-Chief, Chair, President, and CEO

About the Contributors

Medical Editor

Victoria Rand, M.D., is an assistant clinical professor in the Department of Medicine at the University of California at San Francisco. She currently practices at California Pacific Medical Center in San Francisco and she also has a private acupuncture practice. Dr. Rand has lectured widely and received her M.D. with distinction at Cornell University Medical College.

Nutrition Editor

Kathy McManus, M.S., RD, is the director of the Department of Nutrition at Brigham and Women's Hospital. A Harvard teaching affiliate, Ms. McManus is the director of the Nutrition and Behavior Modification Programs for the Program for Weight Management at the Brigham and is coinvestigator on a five-year, NIH-funded obesity study, the POUNDS Lost Trial.

Culinary Editor

Chef Bev Shaffer is the culinary director of "Cooking for Your Heart" at the Section of Cleveland Clinic Preventive Cardiology and Rehabilitation at the Cleveland Clinic Foundation. Her extensive work with this unique outreach program incorporates sound nutrition principles with delicious flavors, educating the public through culinary classes and tastings at Mustard Seed Market in Cleveland, Ohio.

Cholesterol: A Key Factor in the Development of Heart Disease

IF YOU IMAGINE your blood vessels as a superhighway delivering nutrients and oxygen to all the cells in your body, then cholesterol is a proverbial traffic jam. Unfortunately, in this case, lights don't flash and horns don't honk. As the "traffic jam" worsens, pressure builds in the arteries until that telling moment when a plaque breaks off, floating free to the heart or the brain to cause a heart attack or a stroke.

A waxy, fatlike substance that occurs naturally in all parts of the body, some cholesterol is required to ensure normal biological function. It is present in cell walls or membranes everywhere in the body, including the brain, nerves, muscle, skin, liver, intestines, and heart. Your body uses cholesterol to produce many hormones, vitamin D, and the bile acids that help to digest fat. It takes only a small amount of cholesterol in the blood to meet these needs. But when too much cholesterol is present in your bloodstream, the excess is deposited in arteries, including the coronary arteries. As the body's vascular superhighway narrows and blockages (or "traffic jams") form, the signs and symptoms of heart disease surface.

Like any muscle, the heart relies on a constant supply of oxygen and nutrients, which are carried to it by the blood via our vascular superhighway. When the coronary arteries become narrowed or clogged by cholesterol and fat deposits—a process called *atherosclerosis*—and cannot supply enough blood to the heart, the result is coronary heart disease (CHD). If not enough oxygen-carrying blood reaches the heart, you may experience chest pain called *angina*. If the blood supply to a portion of the heart is completely cut off by total blockage of a coronary artery, the result is a heart attack. This is usually due to a sudden closure from a blood clot forming on top of a previous narrowing.

Why Lower Cholesterol Equals a Healthier Heart

Recent studies have shown that lowering cholesterol in people without heart disease greatly reduces their risk for developing coronary heart disease, including heart attacks and CHD-related death. This is true for those with high cholesterol levels and for those with average cholesterol levels. Let's take a look at the evidence.

The Framingham Heart Study established that high blood cholesterol is a risk factor for CHD. Results of this study showed that the higher the cholesterol level, the greater the CHD risk. When cholesterol levels are below 150 milligrams per deciliter (mg/dL), the development of heart disease is rare.

A direct link between high blood cholesterol and CHD has been confirmed by the Lipid Research Clinics Coronary Primary Prevention Trial (in 1984), which showed that lowering total and low-density lipoprotein (LDL—"bad") cholesterol levels significantly reduces CHD.

A 1995 study called the West of Scotland Coronary Prevention Study (WOSCOPS) found that lowering cholesterol reduced the number of heart attacks and deaths from cardiovascular causes in men with high blood cholesterol levels who had not had a heart attack. For five years, more than 6,500 men with total cholesterol levels of 249 mg/dL to 295 mg/dL were given either a cholesterol-lowering drug or a placebo (a dummy pill that looks exactly like the medication), along with a cholesterol-lowering diet. The drug that was given is known as a *statin* (pravastatin), and it reduced total cholesterol levels by 20 percent and LDL cholesterol levels by 26 percent. The study found that in those receiving the statin, the overall risk of having a nonfatal heart attack or dying from CHD was reduced by 31 percent. The need for bypass surgery or angioplasty was reduced by 37 percent, and deaths from all cardiovascular causes were reduced by 32 percent. A very important finding is that deaths from causes other than cardiovascular disease were not increased, and the overall deaths from all causes were reduced by 22 percent.

In 1998, the results of the Air Force/Texas Coronary Atherosclerosis Prevention Study (AFCAPS/TexCAPS) showed that lowering cholesterol in generally healthy people with average cholesterol levels reduced their risk for a first-time major coronary event by 37 percent. Study participants had no obvious evidence of CHD and relatively usual total cholesterol levels (average of 221 mg/dL) and LDL cholesterol levels (average of 150 mg/dL) and lower than usual high-density lipoprotein (HDL—"good") cholesterol levels (average of 36 mg/dL for men and 40 mg/dL for women). This study used a statin drug (lovastatin) along with a low-saturated-fat, low-cholesterol diet to lower cholesterol levels. Study participants who received a placebo followed the same low-saturated-fat, low-cholesterol diet. After one year, total cholesterol levels in the treatment group were lowered by 18 percent and LDL cholesterol levels by 25 percent. The risk for a heart attack was reduced 40 percent, unstable angina 32 percent, the need for bypass surgery or angioplasty 33 percent, and cardio-vascular events 25 percent. The cholesterol-lowering benefits in this study extended to both men and women as well as older adults. There were no significant differences between treatment and placebo groups in non–cardiovascular disease deaths.

Cholesterol Clues: Factors Affecting the Numbers

Your blood cholesterol level is affected not only by what you eat but also by how quickly your body makes LDL cholesterol and disposes of it. In fact, your body makes all the cholesterol it needs, and it is not necessary to take in any additional cholesterol from the foods you eat. There are many factors that help determine whether your LDL cholesterol level is high or low.

Genetics and Cholesterol

Your genes influence how high your LDL cholesterol is by affecting how fast LDL is made and removed from the blood. One specific form of inherited high cholesterol that affects one in five hundred people is *familial hypercholesterolemia*, which often leads to early heart disease. But even if you do not have a specific genetic form of high cholesterol, genes play a role in influencing your LDL cholesterol level.

In Motion: Exercise and the Numbers

Not only will regular physical activity help you to achieve or maintain a healthy weight, but it may also lower LDL cholesterol, raise HDL cholesterol, and reduce blood pressure. Studies also show that exercise may help to reduce levels of triglycerides (a type of fat found in the blood and in foods) and an inflammatory factor called *C-reactive protein* (*CRP*), two additional risk factors involved with heart disease, which we'll discuss later in this chapter.

Age and Gender

Before the age of menopause, women usually have total cholesterol levels that are lower than those of men the same age. As women and men get older, their blood cholesterol levels rise until about sixty to sixty-five years of age. After the age of about fifty, women often have higher total cholesterol levels than men of the same age. Premenopausal women usually have higher HDL (protective) cholesterol levels. After menopause, HDL decreases in many women, increasing their risk for heart disease.

Smoking and Alcohol

Smoking is the number-one risk factor for heart attack. Because smoking reduces HDL cholesterol, which naturally protects against heart disease, women who smoke are at greater risk. In fact, women who smoke have up to six times the risk of heart attack compared to nonsmoking counterparts. Smoking has negative effects not only on cholesterol but also on blood pressure.

Alcohol intake increases HDL cholesterol but does not lower LDL cholesterol. It also thins the blood, reducing the formation of blood clots that block arteries to the heart. Alcohol in moderation is probably good for most people. However, the definition of moderation is tricky, especially for women. The Nurses' Health Study and other studies have shown that two drinks a day increase the risk of developing breast cancer by 20 to 25 percent. Research shows that the increased risk of breast cancer linked to alcohol consumption is seen primarily in women with insufficient levels of folic acid in their diet. This has also been seen among women who develop colon cancer. Experts recommend getting at least 400 micrograms of folic acid a day for those who drink.

Drinking alcohol can also damage the liver and heart muscle, lead to high blood pressure, and raise triglycerides. Because of the risks, alcoholic beverages should not be used as a way to increase HDL levels or prevent heart disease. If you want to get the heart-healthy phytonutrients found in wine, including resveratrol, without consuming alcohol, try red or purple grape juice instead.

Stress and Your Cholesterol

Stress over the long term has been shown in several studies to raise blood cholesterol levels. One way that stress may do this is by affecting people's habits, including the foods they choose. When some people are under stress, they console themselves by eating unhealthy foods. The saturated fat and trans fat in these foods can contribute to higher levels of blood cholesterol. (We'll discuss fats in Chapter 3.) As another coping technique for dealing with stress, people may also smoke or consume alcohol, which as noted earlier can have negative effects on heart disease.

Weight and Your Cholesterol: A Key Factor

Excess weight tends to increase your LDL cholesterol level. If you are overweight and have a high LDL cholesterol level, losing weight may help you lower it. Weight loss also helps to lower triglycerides.

According to the National Heart, Lung, and Blood Institute guidelines, an assessment of being overweight involves three key measures:

❖ Risk factors for diseases and conditions associated with being overweight or obese
❖ Body mass index (BMI)
❖ Waist circumference

Body Mass Index (BMI). The body mass index (BMI) is a measure of your weight relative to your height. Combining BMI with information about your additional risk factors yields your risk for developing obesity-associated diseases. BMI is a reliable indicator of total body fat, which is related to the risk of disease and death. The score is valid for both men and women, but it does have some limits.

❖ It may overestimate body fat in athletes and others who have a muscular build.
❖ It may underestimate body fat in older people and others who have lost muscle mass.
❖ Appropriate weight gain during pregnancy varies and depends upon initial body weight or BMI level. Pregnant women should contact a health professional to ensure appropriate weight gain during pregnancy.

You can use BMI to see whether you are underweight, normal weight, overweight, or obese. Use the body mass index table (Table 1.1) to find your BMI, or you use this equation, taken from the Centers for Disease Control and Prevention:

$$\frac{\text{Weight in pounds}}{\text{Height in inches} \times \text{Height in inches}} \times 703$$

For example, a person who weighs 220 pounds and is 6 feet 3 inches tall has a BMI of 27.5.

TABLE 1.1 **Estimating Your BMI**

Height	Weight (in Pounds)															
	100	110	120	130	140	150	160	170	180	190	200	210	220	230	240	250
5'	20	21	23	25	27	29	31	33	35	37	39	41	43	45	47	49
5'1"	19	21	23	25	26	28	30	32	34	36	38	40	42	43	45	47
5'2"	18	20	22	24	26	27	29	31	33	35	37	38	40	42	44	46
5'3"	18	19	21	23	25	27	28	30	32	34	35	37	39	41	43	44
5'4"	17	19	21	22	24	26	27	29	31	33	34	36	38	39	41	43
5'5"	17	18	20	22	23	25	27	28	30	32	33	35	37	38	40	42
5'6"	16	18	19	21	23	24	26	27	29	31	32	34	36	37	39	40
5'7"	16	17	19	20	22	23	25	27	28	30	31	33	34	36	38	39
5'8"	15	17	18	20	21	23	24	26	27	29	30	32	33	35	36	38
5'9"	15	16	18	19	21	22	24	25	27	28	30	31	32	34	35	37
5'10"	14	16	17	19	20	22	23	24	26	27	29	30	32	33	34	36
5'11"	14	15	17	18	20	21	22	24	25	26	28	29	31	32	33	35
6'	14	15	16	18	19	20	22	23	24	26	27	28	30	31	33	34
6'1"	13	15	16	17	18	20	21	22	24	25	26	28	29	30	32	33
6'2"	13	14	15	17	18	19	21	22	23	24	26	27	28	30	31	32
6'3"	12	14	15	16	17	19	20	21	22	24	25	26	27	29	30	31
6'4"	12	13	15	16	17	18	19	21	22	23	24	26	27	28	29	30

$$\frac{220 \text{ pounds}}{\underset{\text{inches}}{75} \times \underset{\text{inches}}{75}} \times 703 = 27.5$$

To use the body mass index table:

1. Find your height in the left-hand column.
2. Move across in the same row to the number closest to your weight.
3. The number in that column is your BMI. Check your BMI and talk with your doctor to help you achieve a healthy weight.

The BMI score means the following:

* Underweight: Below 18.5
* Normal: 18.5–24.9
* Overweight: 25.0–29.9
* Obesity: 30.0 and above

Waist Circumference: Apples Versus Pears. How you carry your weight is also a factor in the development of heart disease. People who tend to carry weight around their middle (like an apple) are at greater risk for heart disease than those whose weight tends to settle in the hips and thighs (like a pear).

Determine your waist circumference by placing a measuring tape snugly around your waist. It is a good indicator of your abdominal fat, which is another predictor of your risk for developing risk factors for heart disease and other diseases. This risk increases with a waist measurement of more than forty inches in men and more than thirty-five inches in women.

Talk to your doctor to see if you are at an increased risk and if you should lose weight. Your doctor will evaluate your BMI, waist measurement, and other risk factors for heart disease. People who are overweight or obese have a greater chance of developing high blood pressure, high blood cholesterol or other lipid disorders, type 2 diabetes, heart disease, stroke, and certain cancers, and even a small weight loss (just 10 percent of your current weight) will help to lower your risk of developing those diseases.

Cholesterol, Metabolic Syndrome, and Diabetes, Oh My!

Cholesterol doesn't influence just the heart and the vascular system but also has close ties with myriad factors that affect the development of diabetes and metabolic syndrome. Let's take a look.

Diabetes and Cholesterol

Having diabetes increases one's risk for developing heart disease. Because the risk for having a heart attack is typically as high for a person with diabetes as that for a person with heart disease, the LDL goal and cholesterol-lowering treatment are the same as for someone who already has heart disease. Just like for those who have heart disease, the LDL goal is *less than 100 mg/dL*. High triglyceride and low HDL levels are often present in people who have diabetes. After they reach the LDL goal, they should pay attention to the high triglyceride and low HDL levels. We'll discuss the dietary factors influencing all three of the lipoproteins throughout the book, and we'll offer recipes and meal plans to help achieve health goals, deliciously!

Metabolic Syndrome and Cholesterol

The National Cholesterol Education Program has found four health bandits on the loose, collectively defined as metabolic syndrome (aka "insulin resistance syndrome," which was first identified by Dr. Gerald Reaven). Not surprisingly, you'll find cholesterol at the top of the list. The presence of any three of the four of the "Deadly Quartet" indicates foul play (the diagnosis of metabolic syndrome). Let's take a look at the lineup:

* **High levels of triglycerides**—150 mg/dL or higher (we'll discuss these bad guys in Chapter 2)
* **Low levels of HDL cholesterol**—below 40 mg/dL for men and below 50 mg/dL for women (see Chapter 2)
* **Excess weight around the waist**—waist measurement of more than forty inches for men and more than thirty-five inches for women
* **High fasting blood glucose levels**—110 mg/dL or higher
* **High blood pressure**—130/85 mm Hg or higher

According to recent estimates, nearly one in three U.S. adults has high blood pressure, but because there are no symptoms, nearly a third of these people don't even know they have it. In fact, many people have high blood pressure for years without knowing it. Uncontrolled high blood pressure can lead to stroke, heart attack, heart failure, or kidney failure. This is why high blood pressure is often called the "silent killer." The only way to tell if you have high blood pressure is to have your blood pressure checked.

Risk Factors for Metabolic Syndrome. Having one of the bandits lingering means it's likely the others are on their way. That's why it's important that individuals forty-five years or older should consider getting tested for diabetes, especially if they are overweight. In addition, they should consider getting tested if they are younger than forty-five, overweight, and have one or more of the following risk factors:

❖ Family history of diabetes
❖ Low HDL cholesterol and high triglycerides
❖ High blood pressure
❖ History of gestational diabetes (diabetes during pregnancy) or gave birth to a baby weighing more than nine pounds
❖ Minority group background (African American, American Indian, Hispanic American/Latino, or Asian American/Pacific Islander)

Inflammation in Metabolic Syndrome. A number of inflammatory factors and substances in the body—including *C-reactive protein* (*CRP*), *homocysteine*, and *lipoprotein* (*a*)—play a role in the development of heart disease. Not surprisingly, our diet and our weight have a lot to do with increasing or reducing these factors in the body.

Fat cells, or *adipocytes*, are the instruments of inflammation, belting out inflammatory factors including CRP. Because more fat cells are present, being overweight or obese is associated with a state of inflammation. In the past ten years researchers have found these fat-cell-produced compounds are related to insulin resistance, type 2 diabetes, cardiovascular disease, and metabolic syndrome. Dietary fats also play a role in inflammation, which we'll discuss in Chapter 3.

C-reactive protein is so powerful that its presence predicts the risk of cardiovascular disease. This tiny factor is not to be reckoned with. In fact it's even on the American Heart Association's "Most Wanted" list. A recent report published by the American Heart Association/Centers for Disease Control and Prevention (AHA/CDC) duo indicates that CRP measurements may provide important information for assessing heart disease beyond that which may be obtained from established risk factors.

A 2004 study conducted at the Jean Mayer U.S. Department of Agriculture, Human Nutrition Research Center on Aging at Tufts University found that eating more fruits and vegetables significantly lowers levels of C-reactive protein, helping to reduce the risk for heart disease. Studies conducted in 2004 and 2005 at the Centers for Disease Control and Prevention found that diets high in fiber and whole grains also help to reduce CRP. Talk with your doctor about checking your levels of CRP.

Homocysteine, another ally of the Deadly Quartet and an amino acid found normally in the body, also increases your risk of heart disease, stroke, and peripheral vascular disease (a reduced blood flow to the hands and feet).

Numerous studies, including the Physicians' Health Study, the Tromso Study from Norway, the Framingham Heart Study, and a meta-analysis of nearly forty studies, have found that people with elevated levels of homocysteine in their blood are at an increased risk of heart disease.

Scientists have several theories: first, a high level of homocysteine may be involved with the process of atherosclerosis, the gradual buildup of fatty substances in arteries. Homocysteine also may make blood more likely to clot by increasing the stickiness of blood platelets. Clots can block blood flow, causing a heart attack or stroke. Increased homocysteine may affect other substances involved in clotting too. Finally, higher homocysteine levels may make blood vessels less flexible—and so less able to widen to increase blood flow.

Once again, studies have shown that the foods we eat play a role in reducing this obstinate amino acid. Foods rich in folate, vitamin B_6, and vitamin B_{12} actually help to reduce levels of heart-harming homocysteine, reducing the risk for heart disease. Talk with your doctor about getting this checked and let's take a look at some of the "health heroes against homocysteine" that follow.

❖ **Sources of folate.** Black-eyed peas (105 mcg or 25% DV),
cooked spinach (100 mcg or 25% DV), great northern
beans (90 mcg or 20% DV), asparagus (85 mcg or 20%
DV), wheat germ (40 mcg or 10% DV), orange juice (35
mcg or 10% DV), peas (50 mcg or 15% DV), cooked
broccoli (45 mcg or 15% DV), avocados (45 mcg or 10%
DV), and peanuts (40 mcg or 10% DV).

❖ **Sources of vitamin B$_6$.** Potatoes (0.7 mg or 35% DV),
garbanzo beans (0.57mg or 30% DV), chicken breast (0.52
mg or 25% DV), oatmeal (0.42 mg or 20% DV), trout
(0.29 mg or 15% DV), sunflower seeds (0.23 mg or 10%
DV), avocados (0.20 mg or 10% DV), tuna (0.18 mg or
10% DV), and cooked spinach (0.14 mg or 8% DV).

❖ **Sources of vitamin B$_{12}$.** Clams (84.1 mcg or 1,400% DV),
trout (5.4 mcg or 90% DV), salmon (4.9 mcg or 80%
DV), yogurt (1.4 mcg or 25% DV), tuna (1 mcg or 15%
DV), and milk (0.9 mg or 15% DV).

Lipoprotein (a) is a compound in the body that is linked to
LDL cholesterol. Elevated levels of lipoprotein (a) are a risk factor for numerous vascular diseases including heart disease and
stroke. A recent study conducted in 2005 at the Harvard School
of Public Health found that women with levels of lipoprotein (a)
greater than or equal to 30 mg/dL have twice the risk of cardiovascular events as women with lower levels. Scientists have found
that lipoprotein (a) is negatively affected by specific types of
dietary fat, including trans fat and saturated fat (two unhealthy
fats we'll discuss in Chapter 3). Talk with your doctor about getting this checked and reduce levels of lipoprotein to a low by:

❖ Limiting your intake of foods high in saturated fat
❖ Limiting your intake of foods containing trans fats
❖ Choosing good fats from nuts, seeds, nonhydrogenated nut
butters, fish, olive oil, and other expeller pressed oils

A Heart-Smart Diet: The Primary Approach to Reduce Cholesterol

Diet is the first step and the primary therapeutic approach your doctor will recommend to reduce the buildup of plaque. In the past few decades we have gained greater insight into cholesterol and how it is affected by diet. Although cholesterol in foods (like egg yolks and shellfish, for example) can raise cholesterol levels in your body, many other substances—such as trans fat, saturated fat, and refined carbohydrates—also play a role in creating those vascular traffic jams we've been discussing. Plant-based foods—fruits, vegetables, whole grains, legumes, nuts, as well as herbs and spices—conversely, have a protective effect, policing the arteries, ensuring an open road for nutrients and oxygen to travel for optimum health. We will discuss fats, carbohydrates, and nutrients in Chapters 3 and 4 and the heart-helping foods and flavorings in Chapters 5 and 6. Then we'll put it all together in our delicious meal plans and recipes in Chapters 8 and 9, so keep reading!

Focusing on Cholesterol: What the Numbers Mean

KNOWING YOUR CHOLESTEROL score is an important step in taking control of the health of your heart. Once you know the numbers—good or bad—you can take action to reduce your cholesterol and your risk for developing heart disease and other vascular problems. Everyone age twenty and older should have his or her blood cholesterol measured at least once every five years. It is best to have a blood test called a *lipoprotein profile* to find out your cholesterol numbers. This blood test is done after a twelve-hour fast and gives information about the following:

- ❖ Total cholesterol
- ❖ LDL or low-density lipoprotein cholesterol ("bad" cholesterol)
- ❖ HDL or high-density lipoprotein cholesterol ("good" cholesterol)
- ❖ Triglycerides

If it is not possible to have a lipoprotein profile done, knowing your total cholesterol and HDL cholesterol can give you a general idea about your cholesterol levels. If your total cholesterol is

200 mg/dL or more, or if your HDL is less than 40 mg/dL, you will need to have a fasting lipoprotein profile done.

If you do not know your LDL level, you should have it measured. If it does not need specific treatment, you can still take the following steps to keep your cholesterol low and reduce your risk for heart disease:

* Give fruits, vegetables, whole grains, and legumes center stage in your diet.
* Select low-fat, heart-healthy sources of protein such as fish, nuts, soy, and lean poultry.
* Choose the healthy fats over the unhealthy fats (refer to Chapter 3).
* Opt for whole grains over refined foods (see Chapter 3).
* Be physically active.
* Maintain a healthy weight.
* Don't smoke.

Your Total Cholesterol

Total cholesterol is the sum of all the cholesterol in your blood. In general, as you can see from Table 2.1, the higher your total cholesterol, the greater your risk for heart disease. However, some women, particularly athletes, may have a very high HDL (greater than 80) which increases their total cholesterol. Keep in mind that the guidelines are changing, and for patients at high risk, it's not so much total cholesterol, but LDL cholesterol that should be the primary focus.

HDL: The Protective Cholesterol

Approximately one-third to one-fourth of cholesterol in the blood is carried by high-density lipoprotein. This "good" cholesterol has

TABLE 2.1 **Total Cholesterol Levels and Your Risk for Heart Disease**	
Total Cholesterol	**Risk**
Less than 200 mg/dL	Desirable level that puts you at lower risk for heart disease. A cholesterol level of 200 mg/dL or greater increases your risk.
200 to 239 mg/dL	Borderline high.
240 mg/dL and above	High blood cholesterol. A person with this level has more than twice the risk of heart disease compared to someone whose cholesterol is below 200 mg/dL.

the righteous occupation of escorting cholesterol from the blood and back to the liver, where it is processed for elimination from the body. In doing this, HDL makes it less likely that cholesterol in the blood will be deposited in the arteries, creating a vascular backup that can lead to heart disease.

Studies show that levels of HDL are inversely associated with the risk of heart disease. Not only does HDL help sweep cholesterol from the body, but it also protects against heart disease because of its antioxidant and anti-inflammatory action. No wonder it's called the "good cholesterol"! Table 2.2 shows you how HDL affects your risk for heart disease.

Boosting Beneficial Cholesterol

You can boost your heart-helping HDL score by incorporating the healthy carbs and fats into your diet and by opting for a plant-based diet rich in phytonutrients. Exercise also ratchets up your HDL to protect your heart.

TABLE 2.2 **HDL Levels and Your Risk for Heart Disease**	
HDL	**Risk**
Less than 40 mg/dL	A major risk factor for heart disease.
40 to 59 mg/dL	The higher your HDL, the better.
60 mg/dL and above	An HDL of 60 mg/dL and above is considered protective against heart disease.

While consuming a healthy diet and making a habit of exercise helps improve your HDL, a number of other factors can drag it down. Smoking cigarettes, eating a diet high in refined carbohydrates that have been stripped of their nutritious germ and bran layer, consuming trans fats, and taking certain drugs such as beta-blockers, anabolic steroids, and progestational agents (birth control) tend to reduce your good cholesterol.

LDL: Keep It Low

The National Cholesterol Education Program (NCEP) targets low-density lipoprotein as a major culprit of heart disease. LDL carries cholesterol from the liver to the rest of the body. Just as oil and water don't mix, cholesterol, which is fatty, and blood, which is watery, must be packaged into lipoproteins in order to be able to travel in the bloodstream. The cholesterol made in the liver combines with protein, which then carries the cholesterol through the bloodstream.

LDL carries most of the cholesterol in the blood, and the cholesterol from LDL is the main source of damaging buildup and blockage in the arteries. Therefore, the more LDL cholesterol you have in your blood, the greater your risk of heart disease.

While the goals vary for a target LDL based on your personal cardiac risk factors, your LDL level is a good indicator of your risk for heart disease. Lowering LDL is the main goal of treatment if you have high cholesterol. Reducing your LDL, no matter what your age, can help you to protect your heart. It's important to note that for patients with heart disease, the guidelines continue to change. Talk with your doctor regarding your target LDL.

Although diet and exercise play a big role in reducing levels of LDL cholesterol, several other factors come into play and boost your levels of "bad cholesterol," including these:

* Cigarette smoking
* High blood pressure (greater than or equal to 140/90 mm Hg) or taking antihypertensive medication
* Low HDL cholesterol (less than 40 mg/dL)
* Genetics: family history of premature coronary heart disease (CHD in a male relative younger than fifty-five; CHD in a female first-degree relative younger than sixty-five)
* Age (men forty-five or older; women fifty-five or older)

Lipoprotein (a) and LDL

Lipoprotein (a), also known as Lp(a), is a genetic variation of LDL cholesterol, which we briefly discussed in Chapter 1 as a risk factor for vascular diseases. This compound encourages inflammation and fatty deposits in the arteries. Researchers believe that lesions in the walls of arteries contain substances that interact with Lp(a), causing the buildup of fatty deposits. In Chapter 3, we'll discuss how foods, specifically fats in the diet, affect Lp(a).

Your LDL and Therapeutic Lifestyle Changes

The National Heart, Lung, and Blood Institute, part of the National Institutes of Health (nhlbi.nih.gov), has formulated a plan to help reduce LDL cholesterol levels. Coined "Therapeutic Lifestyle Changes (TLC)," this program recommends that people take the following actions:

* Reduce saturated fats to less than 7 percent of total calories (and keep trans fats minimal). Our meal plans and recipes in Chapters 8 and 9 will help you to reach this goal.
* Use the healthy fats in moderation, including polyunsaturated fats, monounsaturated fats, and total fat. Look for cholesterol-cutting plant stanols and sterols, such as canola-based margarine, which we'll discuss in Chapter 3.
* Make carbohydrates (primarily from whole foods such as fruits, vegetables, whole grains, and legumes) the primary source of your total calories.
* Choose lean protein sources.
* Reduce cholesterol-containing foods.
* Get 20 to 30 grams of fiber a day, including increasing the soluble fiber in your diet (to 10 to 25 grams per day).
* Reduce your weight.
* Increase your physical activity.

For specific recommendations on amounts, talk with your doctor and dietitian to create a personal plan to meet your health needs.

Getting enough exercise is up to you, but Healing Gourmet can help you to put these delicious dietary recommendations into practice to reduce your LDL cholesterol and achieve a healthy weight. Our meal plans and recipes in Chapters 8 and 9 help take the guesswork out and put the flavor in. *Eat your heart out!*

When Diet and Exercise Alone Won't Cut It

Some people may have a difficult time reducing LDL cholesterol with diet and exercise alone. Your doctor may prescribe cholesterol-lowering medications, either an over-the-counter one (such as nicotinic acid) or classes of cholesterol-cutters such as statins, fibric acids, or bile acid sequestrants. Be sure to discuss the dangers, side effects, and food and drug interactions of these medications with your doctor.

Triglycerides: Keep It Low

Triglycerides are a form of fat carried through the bloodstream. Most of your body's fat is in the form of triglycerides stored in fat cells (*adipose tissue*), with only a small portion of triglycerides present in the bloodstream.

In general, triglycerides have emerged as an independent risk factor for heart disease. Although high blood triglyceride levels alone do not necessarily cause atherosclerosis (the buildup of cholesterol and fat in the walls of arteries), some lipoproteins that are rich in triglycerides also contain cholesterol, which contributes to atherosclerosis. People with high triglycerides often have high total cholesterol, high LDL cholesterol, and low HDL cholesterol. Table 2.3 illustrates the classifications of triglyceride levels.

TABLE 2.3 **Triglyceride Classifications and Your Risk for Heart Disease**	
Triglyceride	**Risk**
Less than 150 mg/dL	Normal
150 to 199 mg/dL	Borderline high
200 to 499 mg/dL	High
500 mg/dL and above	Very high

Diet does have an effect on triglycerides, but surprisingly, carbohydrates seem to have the most impact. In the next chapter, we discuss how high-glycemic-index carbs appear to increase triglycerides, while some of the healthy fats seem to keep these lipoproteins low. In later chapters, we'll talk about the nutrients and foods with which you should arm yourself for a heart-helping arsenal.

Fats, Carbs, and Your Cholesterol

MIXED MESSAGES ON carbohydrates and fats popularized by some fad diets have led many Americans to make undesirable food choices. Research has shown that the types of fats and carbohydrates we choose have a big impact on cholesterol levels, the development of heart disease, metabolic syndrome, and many other chronic diseases.

Choosing the right fats and carbs has the power to lower total cholesterol, improve our HDL scores, and reduce our LDL and triglyceride levels. Afraid of fat so you skip the olive oil, nuts, and avocados? You're missing out on minerals like magnesium, healthy fats, plus heart-helping antioxidants and phytonutrients! Carb-o-phobic? There go the cholesterol-cutting fiber and heart-helping phytonutrients found abundantly in whole grains and legumes.

Healing Gourmet makes it easy for you to follow the principles discovered by modern science to benefit your heart. In this chapter, we will point out the friends and foes of the fat and carb worlds and how they relate to your cholesterol and risk of associated diseases.

Cholesterol in Food Versus Cholesterol in Your Blood

Although cholesterol in the blood is a factor for heart disease, foods containing cholesterol play only a minor role in the levels that end up in the blood. In fact, in a study of more than eighty thousand female nurses, Harvard researchers found that eating 200 milligrams of cholesterol in food (the equivalent of an egg a day) did not increase the risk for heart disease.

While it's true that egg yolks do contain a lot of cholesterol, they also contain an abundance of protein and nutrients such as vitamins B_{12} and D, folate, riboflavin, and lutein, which may help lower the risk for heart disease.

Unhealthy Fats for Cholesterol

Structurally, fats are simple molecules built around a series of carbon atoms (C) linked to each other in a chain. Dietary fats are composed of long chains containing twelve to twenty-two carbons. A small change in the structure of a dietary fat can make a big impact on your overall health. Let's take a look, first, at the fat foes and their effects on cholesterol levels and the health of your heart.

The Foe: Trans Fat

In nature, most fats occur in what scientists call a "cis" configuration, meaning the hydrogen atoms are on the same side of the double bond. Trans fatty acids, however, are fats produced through a process called *hydrogenation*, which adds a hydrogen to the fat molecule and causes the hydrogen atoms to align on opposite sides of the bond (see Table 3.1). Hydrogenated oil became popular because this type of oil doesn't spoil or become rancid as

TABLE 3.1 Trans Fatty Acids in One Serving of Selected Foods	
Food	**Trans Fatty Acids (Grams per Serving)**
Pound cake	4.3
Microwave popcorn (regular)	2.2
Margarine (stick)	1.8–3.5
Snack crackers	1.8–2.5
Vegetable shortening	1.4–4.2
Vanilla wafers	1.3
Chocolate chip cookies	1.2–2.7
French fries (fast food)	0.7–3.6
Margarine (tub, regular)	0.4–1.6
Doughnuts	0.3–3.8
Salad dressings (regular)	0.06–1.1
White bread	0.06–0.7
Ready-to-eat breakfast cereals	0.05–0.5
Chocolate candies	0.04–2.8
Vegetable oils	0.01–0.06
Snack chips	0–1.2

Fatty acid data from USDA food composition data, 1995

easily as regular oil, and it therefore has a longer shelf life. The more hydrogenated an oil is, the harder it will be at room temperature. For example, a tub of spreadable margarine is less hydrogenated and so has fewer trans fats than a stick of margarine has. Trans fat–free margarines are the best choice.

Most of the trans fats in the American diet are found in commercially prepared baked goods, margarines, snack foods, and processed foods, as well as commercially prepared fried foods, such as french fries, doughnuts, and onion rings. A report from the Institute of Medicine concluded that there is no safe level of trans fats in the diet, which prompted the Food and Drug Administration (FDA) to require that all Nutrition Facts food labels list trans fats by January 1, 2006. Check food labels for "hydrogenated" or "partially hydrogenated" oils: the higher on the list they appear, the more trans fats there are in the product. We'll talk more about understanding the label lingo on foods in Chapter 7.

Recent information from the American Heart Association indicates that heart disease causes about 500,000 deaths annually and is the number-one cause of death in the United States. Therefore, the FDA is proposing to require information on trans fatty acids in nutrition labeling and nutrient content and health claims in response to their importance to public health. Table 3.1 illustrates amounts of trans fats in common foods.

Irrefutably, eating foods containing trans fats increases the risk for heart disease due to the action of these villainous fats on cholesterol. Studies have shown that eating trans fats increases LDL cholesterol while decreasing HDL cholesterol. In fact, the effects of the ratio of LDL to HDL cholesterol are double that of saturated fatty acids, making this fat the most dangerous known to man.

The Nurses' Health Study found that women who ate four teaspoons of stick margarine daily, which deliver 1.8 to 3.5 grams of this unhealthy fat, had a 50 percent greater risk of heart disease than women who ate margarine only rarely.

In addition, seven recent studies compared the effects of trans fats to their naturally occurring counterparts. These studies showed that trans fats increase triglycerides compared with other fats.

The Nurses' Health Study evaluated 823 women for markers of inflammation and found that eating trans fat–containing foods increases C-reactive protein, an inflammatory factor most associated with heart disease and diabetes.

Additionally, nine out of ten trials showed that these unhealthy fats also increase levels of lipoprotein (a). Elevated levels of this inflammatory factor increase the risk for numerous vascular diseases including heart disease and stroke.

 Healing Tip

While the FDA is requiring food manufacturers to provide more information on the trans fat content of foods, you can sleuth out hidden trans fat by looking for "partially hydrogenated oils" or "vegetable shortening" on food labels to help reduce your cholesterol and the risk for heart disease, diabetes, and metabolic syndrome. Choose trans fat–free shortenings and baked goods.

The Foe: Saturated Fat

Saturated fats are mainly animal fats. The major sources are red meat, whole-milk dairy products (cheese, milk, and ice cream), poultry skin, and egg yolks. Some plant foods are also high in saturated fats, including coconut and coconut oil, palm oil, and palm kernel oil. With saturated fatty acids, each of the interior carbon atoms is bonded to two hydrogen atoms as well as two other carbons. All of the bonds available for hydrogen are filled or "saturated" with hydrogen, hence the name.

It is a long-known fact that saturated fats increase levels of total cholesterol (both LDL and HDL), as well as triglycerides. Sixteen populations in seven countries were observed for the types of fats they consumed and the risk of heart disease. Researchers found that saturated fats in the diet are undeniably linked to the risk of heart disease. Saturated fats also have negative effects on insulin function. As we consume saturated fats, they are stored in cells as triglycerides, causing damage to those cells.

Saturated fats have been found to increase levels of lipoprotein (a) (discussed in Chapter 1), an inflammatory factor that increases the risk for numerous vascular diseases including heart disease and stroke.

 Healing Tip

Opt for plant-based fats, fish, low-fat dairy, and lean poultry instead of red meat, processed meat, and full-fat dairy products to reduce heart-harming saturated fat in your diet.

Healthy Fats for Cholesterol

Eating the right fats helps to boost your HDL and reduce LDL and inflammatory factors associated with the development of heart disease and its negative associates (including metabolic syndrome). Let's take a look at the delicious, plant-based fats to enjoy for a healthy heart.

The Friend: Monounsaturated Fat

Monounsaturated fats (MUFAs) are derived from vegetable sources including olives, nuts, and avocados. Monounsaturated fats have a double bond that allows the fatty acid chain to be a bit more fluid, making them liquid at room temperature. Monounsaturated fats are best known for their ability to lower LDL and raise HDL cholesterol levels if part of a healthful diet, and they have also been found to help keep blood sugar stable. Evidence from the Mediterranean diet also supports this research, showing that consumption of MUFA-rich olive oil helps to reduce inflammatory processes and reduce heart disease risk.

In addition, foods containing MUFAs also contain a spectrum of heart-helping phytonutrients such as phenols, beta-sitosterol, and lutein to ally forces. (In Chapter 5, we discuss how compounds in foods team up to protect our health, a phenomenon called "synergy.")

 Healing Tip

Stock your pantry with nuts, peanut butter, trans fat–free butters, olive oil, canola oil, and avocados to enjoy the benefits of health-promoting MUFAs. Trade in your chips and pretzels for a MUFA-rich snack mix including popcorn popped in canola oil and raw almonds.

The Friend: Polyunsaturated Fat

The human body needs fatty acids and can make all but two of them: linolenic and linoleic acid. These fats must be supplied by the diet, hence the term "essential fatty acids." Used by the body to maintain cell membranes and make hormonelike substances that regulate blood pressure, clotting, immune response, insulin function, and blood lipids, the polyunsaturated fat (PUFA) side of the fat family gets special treatment for its positive impact on the health of the heart. Like their friendly cousins, the monounsaturated fats, PUFAs are best known for their ability to lower LDL and raise HDL cholesterol levels when part of a healthful diet.

A 2005 study conducted at the Department of Nutrition of the Harvard School of Public Health evaluated the role of specific fats and the risk of heart disease among 78,778 women who were free of heart disease and diabetes. Researchers found an inverse relationship between PUFAs in the diet and the risk of heart disease, particularly among younger or overweight women.

Let's take a look at each of the essentials and their role in cholesterol levels and heart disease risk.

Omega-3 Fatty Acids. *Omega-3 fatty acids,* also known as *linolenic acid,* are essential fatty acids (EFAs) that come from both plant and animal sources. Given linolenic acid, the body can make *eicosapentaenoic acid (EPA)* and *docosahexaenoic acid (DHA),* the two major fatty acids in fish. The greatest amounts of EPA and DHA are found in oily, dark-fleshed fish, such as tuna, bluefish, and salmon, that live in deep, cold waters. *Alpha-linolenic acid* is the other essential fatty acid and is found most abundantly in canola oil. It is also found in flaxseed and walnuts. Soybeans also contain a balance of omega-3 fats.

Numerous studies have shown that people who eat omega-3-rich foods have lower rates of heart disease, and scientists are beginning to discover why. From reducing LDL cholesterol and C-reactive protein to boosting HDL, there are plenty of reasons that fish is really good for the heart.

A 2005 study published in *Atherosclerosis* found that omega-3 fatty acids in the diet have a positive association with HDL cholesterol levels in men, suggesting this boost in the good cholesterol may be to credit for the heart-protecting benefits.

These good fats may also protect against the development of heart disease in women with diabetes. A 2003 Harvard study followed 5,103 female nurses diagnosed with diabetes and found that the women eating the most omega-3-rich fish had the lowest risk of heart disease.

A 2004 study published in the *Journal of Nutrition* found that omega-3 fats help to reduce inflammatory factors—including C-reactive protein. In fact, women getting the most omega-3s in their diet had 29 percent lower levels of CRP.

Omega-6 Fatty Acids. *Omega-6 fatty acids,* also known as *linoleic acid,* are much more common in the American diet and are found in soybean oil, safflower oil, sunflower oil, corn oil, wheat germ, sesame, as well as red and processed meats. Omega-6 fatty acids have potent cholesterol-lowering effects. However, while omega-6 fatty acids are an important part of the heart-helping team of PUFAs, science is showing that there is a delicate balance when it comes to these "healthy fats" and that these health heroes may also have a dark side.

Researchers postulate that because omega-6 fatty acids are more readily available and consumed in Western countries, and because our Paleolithic ancestors consumed a balance of omega-3 to omega-6 fatty acids, an imbalance could negatively influence inflammatory processes associated with heart disease. Some studies show that excess omega-6s can promote some inflammatory factors. The proper ratio of omega-3 to omega-6 in our diet should be two-to-one to get the maximum health benefits from the PUFAs. Thus, while PUFAs should make up a good part of the fats in your diet, be sure to balance your sixes with your threes.

 Kitchen Prescription

To improve your ratio of omega-3 fatty acids to omega-6 fatty acids, take these steps:

+ Choose canola oil as one of your oils when cooking.
+ Balance the selection of nuts as a snack and choose walnuts as a source of omega-3 fats.
+ Look for new food products with enhanced omega-3s, including eggs, breads, and cereals.
+ Try ground flaxseed meal or hempseed meal as an addition to smoothies, cereals, and baked goods.
+ Include cold-water fish, such as salmon and tuna, in your diet.

The Dish on Fish and Mercury. Although there is no doubt that including fish in your diet will deliver protective essential fatty acids and B vitamins, research shows that certain types of fish may contain dangerous levels of mercury. Nearly all fish and shellfish contain traces of *methylmercury*, a type of mercury found in water that can be harmful, especially to unborn babies and young children whose nervous systems are still developing. The risk from mercury lies in both the type of seafood consumed and the amount. The Food and Drug Administration and the Environmental Protection Agency (EPA) through a joint consumer advisory warn that women who may be trying to become pregnant, pregnant women, nursing mothers, and young children should avoid the types of fish and shellfish with higher levels of mercury and eat only those that have lower levels. If you regularly eat types of fish high in methylmercury, the substance can accumulate in your blood over time. Although it is removed from the body naturally, it may take more than a year for the levels to drop significantly, which is why even women who are trying to become pregnant should avoid eating certain types of fish.

While almost all fish and shellfish contain traces of methylmercury, larger fish that have lived longer contain the highest levels of methylmercury, as it accumulates over time. Avoid eating shark, swordfish, or king mackerel because they contain high levels of mercury and pose the greatest risk. You should be eating up to 12 ounces (two average meals) a week of a variety of fish and shellfish that are lower in mercury. We offer several recipes incorporating fish in Chapter 9. Four of the most commonly eaten fish that are low in mercury are shrimp, canned light tuna, salmon, and catfish. Albacore (white) tuna has more mercury than canned light tuna. When choosing your meals of fish and shellfish, you may eat up to six ounces (one average meal) of albacore tuna per week. In addition, you should check to see if advisories exist concerning the safety of fish caught in local lakes, rivers, and coastal areas. If no advice is available, eat up to six ounces per week of fish you catch from local waters, but don't consume any other fish during that week.

Not All Carbs Are Created Equal

Carbohydrates are produced by photosynthesis in plants and are the primary source of immediate and time-released energy found in plant foods including fruits, vegetables, grains, legumes, and tubers. Carbohydrates have an important role in the functioning of the internal organs, nervous system, and muscles and are the best source of energy for endurance athletics because they provide both immediate and time-released energy. These compounds are needed to regulate protein and fat metabolism as well as to help to fight infections, promote growth, and lubricate the joints.

At one time, carbs were grouped into two main categories. Simple carbs included sugars such as fruit sugar (fructose), corn or grape sugar (dextrose or glucose), and table sugar (sucrose); complex carbs included everything made of three or more linked sugars. In the digestive system, carbohydrates are broken down into single sugar molecules, which are then absorbed into the bloodstream and used as energy. Evidence shows that carb choices have a big impact on inflammation and blood sugar and cholesterol levels, all of which affect our risk for heart disease.

Traditionally, it has been assumed that complex carbohydrates cause smaller rises in blood sugar than do simple carbohydrates. However, a growing body of evidence contradicts this notion. In fact, white bread and potatoes are digested almost immediately and converted to glucose, causing blood sugar to rapidly spike—refuting the theory that complex carbohydrates are different from simple sugars in terms of their effects on blood sugar levels.

Glycemic Index Versus Glycemic Load

A new system that has been embraced by many in the scientific community called the *glycemic index* (*GI*) rates foods according to how fast and how far they push blood sugar. This system gives us a better indication of how carb-rich foods affect health. It has been shown that the GI of a food depends on the speed of digestion and absorption into the body, which is largely determined by both its physical and chemical properties. Typically, foods with less starch to gelatinize—such as pasta—and those containing a high level of soluble fiber—such as whole-grain barley, oats, and rye—have slower rates of digestion and lower GI values. Another important factor of GI values is the ratio of a compound called *amylose* to a fiber called *amylopectin*. Foods with a higher amylose/amylopectin ratio—such as legumes and parboiled (quick-cooking) rice—tend to have lower GI values, because of the compact structure of amylose, which blunts the effects of enzymatic reactions. Conversely, amylopectin is a branched compound, making it more available to enzymatic attack in the body, promoting digestion. Use of the GI has shown that many complex carbohydrates (such as white bread and potatoes) cause endocrine responses that rival pure glucose, further casting doubt on the usefulness of the simple versus complex classification system.

The principal argument against the GI concept is that it cannot tell the entire story, as blood sugar levels are influenced by both the quantity and the quality (GI rating) of the carbohydrate. In response to this concern, the concept of *glycemic load* (*GL*) was introduced. Defined as the product of the GI value of a food and its carbohydrate content, GL incorporates both the quality and quantity of carbohydrate consumed.

With white bread (or glucose) used as the reference standard for glycemic load, dietary GL quantifies the glucose-raising potential of dietary carbohydrates, with each unit of dietary GL representing the equivalent glycemic effect of 1 gram of carbohydrate from white bread. In general, carbohydrate-dense foods with low fiber content, including potatoes, refined cereal products, and many sugar-sweetened beverages, have high GI and GL values; whereas whole grains, fruits, and vegetables with high fiber content provide low to very low GLs per serving. It should be noted, however, that many low-GI foods are not necessarily high in fiber (e.g., pasta, converted rice, and dairy products), whereas some high-fiber whole-meal bread and cereal products (such as instant oatmeal) are high in GI.

Valuable research in recent years has offered additional insight into how carbohydrates affect the endocrine system, insulin production, inflammatory processes, hunger, overeating, weight gain, and heart disease. While the glycemic index is an important tool that has provided insight, research is ongoing.

Refined Versus Whole Carbohydrates: Messing with Mother Nature

You may be familiar with complex versus simple carbs, but science has now moved toward classifying carbohydrates as either "whole" or "refined." When it became a common practice to refine the wheat flour for bread by milling it and discarding the bran and germ, consumers lost myriad health-protective nutrients. In the 1940s, Congress passed legislation requiring that all grain products that cross state lines be enriched with iron, thiamin, riboflavin, and niacin. In 1996, this legislation was amended to include folate, due to its important role in preventing birth defects. Although enrichment—the process of adding nutrients to a food to meet a specific standard—restores and raises many of the nutrients lost during refining, recent research shows that the health consequences cannot be compensated for by adding individual nutrients back to a refined grain product for several reasons.

First, by removing the germ and bran layers of a grain, a naturally low-GI food is turned into a high-GI one. The fibrous coating serves to slow digestion, keeping blood sugar on an even keel. Also, the surface area is increased with refined grain products, enhancing digestive enzyme processes.

Second, many nutrients in the germ and bran layers are not added back to the refined grain product, or the body poorly absorbs them. This is especially true of minerals, which are not as well absorbed from enriched foods as from naturally occurring sources.

Third, the "new nutritional frontier" is still in its infancy, and we have yet to identify all of the health-protective compounds in every food. When we alter a food from its natural state—by refining, for example—we may be removing a cocktail of phytonutrients and other compounds that protect us from disease.

Refined carbs, which are stripped of their virtuous germ and bran layers, give a bad name to a good food group. The naked truth of the matter is that when the integrity of whole grains is preserved, the effects on health are nothing short of wholesome.

How Carbohydrate Choices Affect Your Heart and Your Cholesterol Levels

With all this talk about insulin and blood sugar, you may be asking yourself, "What does this have to do with cholesterol and my risk of heart disease?" The answer is *everything*! Large studies have proved that blood sugar is an independent predictor of heart disease in people without diabetes. The glycemic index and glycemic load are associated with risk factors of heart disease including HDL cholesterol, triglycerides, and C-reactive protein, not to mention weight gain.

High-glycemic-index and high-glycemic-load foods are associated with lower levels of HDL cholesterol and elevated triglycerides, both risk factors for heart disease.

A 2002 study published in *Diabetes Care* evaluated the effects of a low-GI diet on lipids and body fat in men without diabetes. The study found that after five weeks, the low-GI diet had reduced cholesterol levels, lipoproteins, and body fat, helping to lower the risk for heart disease.

The Third National Health and Nutrition Examination Survey used information from 13,907 participants to determine the effects of high-glycemic-index and high-glycemic-load foods on HDL cholesterol levels. The study found that eating high-GI and high-GL foods reduced levels of heart-healthy HDL among participants.

Similarly, the Nurses' Health Study evaluated GI and GL for their effects on triglyceride levels in women who had gone through menopause. The study found that a high-GL diet is a factor in the development of heart disease, particularly among women who are prone to insulin resistance.

Carbohydrate Choices and Inflammation

In Chapter 1 we discussed some of the inflammatory factors that play a role in the development of heart disease. Recent research has shown that the types of carbohydrates we choose have an impact on increasing or decreasing these heart-harming factors. Let's take a look at the research.

High-glycemic-load foods have been found to increase levels of C-reactive protein in women. A 2005 article in *Med Hypotheses* reports that women who adopted a low-GL, whole-food, vegan diet rich in soluble fiber saw a 28 percent reduction in levels of CRP. (Learn more about fiber on page 44.)

A 2004 study published in *JAMA* evaluated different diets and their effects on overweight or obese young adults (aged eighteen to forty). At the end of the study, the participants on the low-glycemic-load diet reported lower levels of C-reactive protein, reduced triglycerides and blood pressure, as well as less hunger.

Carbohydrate Choices and Your Weight

As mentioned in Chapter 1, excess weight tends to increase your LDL cholesterol level. Almost every study conducted on the effects of carbohydrates on appetite has shown that low-GI/GL foods produce a feeling of satiety, or satisfaction, for a longer period of time than do their high-GI/GL counterparts. Thus, your carbohydrate choices can factor into controlling your weight and keeping your cholesterol levels in check.

In addition, because of their high fiber and water content, whole-grain foods contain fewer calories gram for gram than the same amount of corresponding refined grain foods. The Nurses' Health Study showed that women with the greatest increased intake of whole grains gained an average of 1.52 kilograms less than did those with the smallest increase in intake of whole-grain foods. In addition, women with the highest consumption of whole grains had a 49 percent lower risk of major weight gain than did women with the highest consumption of refined grains. Researchers believe that the insulin-elevating effects of high-GI foods promote weight gain by directing nutrients away from use in muscles and toward storage in fat cells.

Carbs in the Kitchen

Now that we've set the stage for understanding how carbohydrates affect your cholesterol and risk for heart disease, let's put that knowledge into practice! While certain fruits, such as watermelon and carrots, are high on the GI scale (as seen in Table 3.2), they should not be avoided because of their abundance of phytonutrients, fiber, and other nutrients. However, aim to stock your pantry with moderate-GI (Table 3.3) and low-GI foods (Table 3.4) and enjoy them often. We'll show you how easy it is to clean up your carb act and give you practical pairings to get your healthy carbs and healthy fats, deliciously.

Small changes can make a big impact on your health. The list that starts on page 42 offers some helpful suggestions for replacing the carbs higher on the glycemic index with some lower-GI alternatives.

TABLE 3.2 **High-GI Foods (>69)**	
Product	**Food**
Breads and bakery	White bread
	Whole-meal bread
	Pretzels
	French bread
Breakfast cereals	Cornflakes
	Rice Krispies
	Cheerios
Confectionery	Jelly beans
	Life Savers
	Skittles
Fruits and vegetables	Carrots
	Watermelon
	Potatoes
	Parsnips
Rice, grains, and pastas	Low-amylase rice

TABLE 3.3 Moderate-GI Foods (55–69)

Product	Food
Breads and bakery	Sourdough
	Pita bread
	Barley bread
	Rye bread
	Whole-wheat bread
Breakfast cereals	Quick-cooking oatmeal
	Cream of wheat
	Muesli
Dairy foods	Ice cream, full-fat
Fruits and vegetables	Pineapple
	Banana
Rice, grains, and pastas	Brown rice
	Linguine
	White rice
	Popcorn

❖ Instead of white bread, try pumpernickel or dark, whole-grain breads. Pepperidge Farm Whole Grain breads are an excellent choice, providing whole grains and no trans fats.

❖ Instead of white rice, try basmati rice or Lundberg rice, converted rice, or couscous.

❖ Instead of sugary breakfast cereal, try muesli, steel-cut oats, bran cereal, or one of Kashi's delicious whole-grain, high-fiber, high-protein cereals. We like Kashi's Heart to Heart products for their soluble fiber, antioxidants, B-vitamins, and whole grains, of course.

TABLE 3.4 Low-GI Foods (<55)

Product	Food
Breads and bakery	Pumpernickel
	Heavy mixed grain
Breakfast cereals	All Bran
	Toasted muesli
	Psyllium-based cereal
	Oatmeal (old-fashioned)
Dairy foods	Milk, full-fat
	Soy milk
	Milk, skim
	Yogurt, low-fat, fruit
Fruits and vegetables	Grapefruit
	Peaches
	Apples
	Pears
	Oranges
	Grapes
	Kiwi
	Sweet potatoes
Rice, grains, and pastas	Fettuccini
	Whole-wheat spaghetti
	Spaghetti
	Long-grain rice
	Bulgur
Legumes	Peanuts
	Soybeans
	Lentils
	Chickpeas
	Baked beans (canned)

❖ Instead of potatoes, try beans or whole-grain pasta. We like multigrain Barilla PLUS, which also provides protein, fiber and omega-3 fats.
❖ Instead of white crackers, try whole-grain rye or whole-wheat crackers. Try Ryvita whole-grain crackers.
❖ Instead of cakes, light muffins, or pastry, try bran muffins or use whole-grain mixes.

In addition, here are some suggestions from Healing Gourmet of foods that will give you a daily dose of those good fats and good carbs, with no sacrifice on taste. For more ideas, see the recipe and meal-planning sections, and visit our website, healing gourmet.com.

❖ Pepperidge Farm German Dark Wheat bread with all-natural peanut butter for whole grains, PUFAs, and low-GI legumes
❖ Ryvita Dark Rye Crackers and hummus for whole grains, low-GI legumes, and MUFAs
❖ Grilled wild salmon and Lundberg Wehani Rice for omega-3s and whole grains
❖ Stonyfield Farms black cherry yogurt and ground flax for low-GI carbs and omega-3s

Feast on Fiber: Bulk Is Better

One of the heart-helping properties of whole-grain, carbohydrate-rich foods is their abundance of fiber, an important nonnutritive compound that helps to sweep cholesterol out of the body and keep blood sugar on an even keel.

There are two general categories of fiber: soluble and insoluble. Soluble fibers, which are easily digested, can be divided into three major types: *pectins* (found in root vegetables, cabbage, apples, whole-wheat bran, and beans), *gums* (which can be obtained from oatmeal, dried beans, and other legumes), and *mucilages* (which are synthesized by plant cells and are found in food additives).

There are also several types of insoluble fibers. One is *cellulose*, which can be found in cabbage, peas, apples, root vegetables, whole-wheat flour, beans, bran, and wheat. Another is *hemicellulose*, which is found in bran, cereals, and whole grains. *Lignan*, found most abundantly in flaxseed, is a phytonutrient that works very much like an insoluble fiber. Fiber is actually classified as a carbohydrate. (In the United States, the total carbohydrates listed on a food label will include dietary fiber, although the fiber is listed separately.) Insoluble fiber is important to regulate gastrointestinal functions and to keep the colon clean.

Research studies confirm, and it is the position of the American Dietetic Association, that fiber is an important element in reducing cholesterol and preventing cardiovascular disease. Water-soluble fiber, in particular, is beneficial for people concerned with lowering cholesterol levels and preventing heart disease for several key reasons.

* It soaks up excess bile acids found in the intestinal tract, which are converted into blood cholesterol by the body.
* It delays stomach emptying, causing a feeling of fullness or satiety that is useful in achieving or maintaining a healthy weight.

Fiber, Heart Disease, and C-Reactive Protein

A Harvard study found that weight gain among 74,091 nurses was inversely associated with high-fiber, whole-grain foods and positively associated with the intake of refined-grain foods. Getting lots of dietary fiber has also been linked to a lower risk of heart disease in a number of large studies that followed people for many years. In a Harvard study of more than forty thousand male health professionals, researchers found that a high total dietary fiber intake was linked to a 40 percent lower risk of coronary heart disease, compared to a low fiber intake. In the Nurses' Health Study, which involved nearly sixty-nine thousand women in a ten-year follow-up investigation, researchers found that fiber obtained from eating cereals, vegetables, and fruit lowered CHD risk. Increased consumption of cereal grains conferred the greatest benefit.

In addition, a recent study conducted at the Centers for Disease Control and Prevention examined the association between dietary fiber and serum concentration of C-reactive protein. Using data from the National Health and Nutrition Examination Survey 1999–2000, which evaluated the diets of 3,920 participants, the study concluded that dietary fiber intake was inversely associated with serum CRP concentration.

Getting Fiber into Your Diet

The American Diabetes Association (ADA) recommends 20 to 35 grams of fiber daily for all adults. The Therapeutic Lifestyle Changes (TLC) program suggests that people with high cholesterol levels can benefit from 10 to 25 grams of *soluble* fiber daily. Not all labels separate fiber into soluble and insoluble, so it's important to eat a wide variety of fiber-rich foods to get a good balance. In Table 3.5 we summarize sources of fiber.

* Choose fresh fruits or vegetables rather than juice.
* Eat the skin and membranes of cleaned fruits and vegetables.
* Choose bran and whole-grain breads and cereals daily.

TABLE 3.5 Fiber Content of Selected Foods

Food Item	Total(g)	Soluble(g)	Insoluble(g)
Legumes			
Pinto beans (½ cup, cooked)	7.4	1.9	5.5
Chickpeas (½ cup)	6.2	1.3	4.9
Kidney beans (½ cup, cooked)	5.8	2.9	2.9
Navy beans (½ cup, cooked)	5.8	2.2	3.6
Northern beans (½ cup)	5.6	1.4	4.2
Soybeans (½ cup, cooked)	5.1	2.3	2.8
Tofu (½ cup)	1.4	0.9	0.6
Cereal Grains			
Barley (½ cup, cooked)	4.2	0.9	3.3
Millet (½ cup, cooked)	3.3	0.6	2.7
Bulgur (½ cup, cooked)	2.9	0.5	2.4
Noodles (whole-wheat)	2.3	0.5	1.8
Rice, brown (½ cup, cooked)	1.7	0.1	1.6
Rice, wild (½ cup, cooked)	1.5	0.2	1.3

(continued)

TABLE 3.5 *(continued)*

Food Item	Total(g)	Soluble(g)	Insoluble(g)
Cereal Grains *(continued)*			
Couscous (½ cup, cooked)	1.3	0.3	1.0
Noodles (white spaghetti)	0.9	0.4	0.5
Noodles (spinach, ½ cup)	0.9	0.4	0.5
Rice, white (½ cup, cooked)	0.2	0	0.2
Breads (1 medium slice)			
Pita (7″ diameter, wheat)	4.4	0.7	3.7
Whole-wheat	1.9	0.3	1.6
Multigrain	1.8	0.3	1.5
Pumpernickel	1.5	0.8	0.7
Rye	1.5	0.8	0.7
Tortilla (6″ diameter, plain)	1.4	0.2	1.1
Tortilla (8″ diameter, plain)	1.4	0.4	1.0
White or sourdough	0.7	0.4	0.3

Cereal (1 cup)			
All Bran	10.0	1.0	9.0
Raisin Bran	8.4	1.2	7.2
Oatmeal	3.8	1.8	2.0
Cheerios	2.6	1.2	1.4
Farina	1.2	0.5	0.7
Cornflakes	0.7	0	0.7
Grits, corn	0.4	0	0.4
Snacks			
Popcorn (microwave, 3 cups)	2.4	0	2.4
Popcorn (light, 3 cups)	2.3	0	2.3
Fruits (fresh)			
Apple (3″ diameter)	5.7	1.5	4.2
Figs (3 small)	5.3	2.3	3.0
Orange (3″ diameter)	4.4	2.6	1.8
Raspberries (½ cup)	4.2	0.4	3.8
Pear (3″ diameter)	4.0	2.2	1.8

(continued)

TABLE 3.5 *(continued)*

Food Item	Total(g)	Soluble(g)	Insoluble(g)
Fruits (fresh) (continued)			
Blackberries (½ cup)	3.8	3.1	0.7
Mango (medium)	3.7	1.5	2.2
Peach (medium)	3.2	1.3	1.9
Kiwi (large)	3.1	0.7	2.4
Banana (7″ long)	2.8	0.7	2.1
Prunes (3 medium)	1.9	1.0	0.9
Blueberries (½ cup)	1.9	0.2	1.7
Strawberries (½ cup)	1.9	0.5	1.4
Plum (large)	1.7	0.9	0.8
Cherries (½ cup, fresh)	1.7	0.5	1.2
Applesauce (½ cup)	1.6	0.5	1.1
Raisins (¼ cup)	1.5	0.4	1.1
Grapefruit (half, 4″ diameter)	1.5	1.2	0.3
Pineapple (½ cup)	1.0	0.1	0.9
Grapes (½ cup)	0.8	0.3	0.5
Melon (⅕ of 6″ diameter)	0.7	0.2	0.5

Juice (orange, 6 oz)	0.4	0.2	0.2
Juice (apple, 6 oz)	0.2	0.1	0.1
Vegetables			
Artichoke (medium, cooked)	6.5	4.7	1.8
Brussels sprouts (½ cup)	3.3	2.0	1.3
Jicama (raw, ½ cup)	3.2	1.7	1.5
Chiles (hot pepper, raw)	3.0	1.5	1.5
Carrots (baby, 6)	2.8	1.4	1.4
Corn (½ cup)	2.0	0.3	1.7
Beans (cooked, ½ cup)	1.9	0.8	1.1
Cabbage (green, cooked)	1.8	0.8	1.0
Cauliflower (½ cup)	1.7	0.4	1.3
Carrots (cooked, ½ cup)	1.6	1.1	1.5
Beets (½ cup)	1.5	0.7	0.8
Asparagus spears (cooked)	1.4	0.7	0.7
Bok choy (½ cup)	1.4	0.5	0.9
Broccoli (cooked)	1.4	1.2	1.2
Eggplant, cooked (½ cup)	1.3	0.4	0.9

(continued)

TABLE 3.5 *(continued)*

Food Item	Total(g)	Soluble(g)	Insoluble(g)
Vegetables *(continued)*			
Broccoli (raw, ½ cup)	1.3	0.5	0.8
Cauliflower (raw, ½ cup)	1.3	0.5	0.8
Celery (1 large stalk)	1.1	0.4	0.7
Lettuce (Romaine, 1 cup)	0.9	0.3	0.6
Lettuce (Iceberg, 1 cup)	0.8	0.1	0.7
Cabbage (red, shredded)	0.8	0.3	0.5
Greens (cooked, ½ cup)	0.4	0.1	0.
Frozen and mixed vegetables (½ cup)			
Lima beans/corn	4.9	1.8	3.1
Peas (cooked, ½ cup)	4.3	1.2	3.1
Corn/green beans/carrots	4.0	1.9	2.1
Sweet potatoes (½ cup)	3.8	1.4	2.4
Pumpkin (mashed, ½ cup)	3.6	0.5	3.1
Squash (winter, ½ cup cooked)	3.3	1.9	1.4
Potato (w/skin, medium)	2.9	1.2	1.7

Spinach (cooked, ½ cup)	2.7	0.5	2.2
Peas/carrots	2.5	0.9	1.6
Onions (cooked, ½ cup)	2.0	1.2	0.8
Broccoli/peppers/mushroom	1.8	0.7	1.1
Mushrooms (cooked, sliced)	1.8	0.2	1.6
Squash (butternut, ½)	1.7	0.7	1.0
Potato (mashed, ½ cup)	1.6	0.9	0.7
Broccoli/cauliflower	1.5	0.6	0.9
Peppers (green/red, ½ cup)	1.3	0.5	0.8
Water chestnuts (½ cup)	1.2	0.9	1.3
Zucchini (cooked, ½ cup)	1.2	0.5	0.7
Tomatoes (medium, raw)	0.9	0	0.9
Spinach (raw, 1 cup)	0.4	0.1	0.3

❖ When you increase fiber, you should also increase your water intake.

❖ Eat fewer processed foods and more fresh ones, as processing often removes fiber.

❖ Try to get fiber from foods rather than fiber supplements, as foods are more nutritious and supply an array of health-promoting phytonutrients.

Love Your Legumes

The evidence that beans reduce cholesterol and protect against heart disease is so strong that we're devoting a section to get you to *love your legumes*! Beans are a low-glycemic food and an excellent source of fiber, making them a smart choice for people concerned with weight control and heart disease.

Beans release sugar slowly into the bloodstream ensuring blood sugar stays stable. The insoluble fiber in beans causes the body to produce more insulin receptor sites—tiny "docks" that insulin molecules latch onto—meaning more insulin gets into cells where it is needed, and less is present in the bloodstream where it can cause problems. The low glycemic index of beans has been attributed to many factors including their fiber, tannin, and phytic acid contents. Beans also help to keep cholesterol low, thanks to compounds including saponins and phytoestrogens.

Saponins are naturally occurring compounds found in legumes. These compounds combine with lipids and form soap-like foams that carry cholesterol out of the body. Saponins decrease blood lipids, lower cancer risks, and reduce blood sugar.

Phytoestrogens, including *isoflavones* found primarily in soybeans, have been found to reduce cholesterol and improve glucose control and insulin resistance. Researchers believe these compounds modulate the secretion of insulin from the pancreas and also act as antioxidants.

Kitchen Prescription

Try our N'Orleans Red Beans and Rice recipe in Chapter 9 for a delicious Bayou-style garden entrée that fills you up without weighing you down. In the mood for something zesty? Try our Caribbean Black Beans and Rice instead. Bean up!

Now that you have some ideas for balancing the good and bad fats and carbohydrates, plus getting a healthy dose of fiber and learning to love your legumes, it's time to look at the benefits of increasing your intake of antioxidants and phytonutrients, as well as ways to incorporate these important foods into your heart-healthy diet.

4

Antioxidants, Phytonutrients, and Other Cholesterol-Lowering Nutrients

ALONG WITH VITAMINS and minerals that help to protect against heart disease, thousands of phytonutrients in foods are getting special attention for their honorable actions as defenders of our health. Each with its own unique role, these compounds work together to keep cholesterol levels in check and reduce the risk for heart disease. In this chapter we'll discuss the lineup of cholesterol-reducing nutrients and their position in preventing cardiovascular disease.

Free Radical Defense

Free radicals make about ten thousand attacks on the cells in our body every day. These unstable oxygen molecules have lost an electron and—like a sneaky opponent—move swiftly through the playing field of your body, trying to steal electrons from other molecules. This in turn creates more free radicals and leaves damaged cells in the wake. Some free radicals arise normally during metabolism, but environmental factors such as pollution, poor food choices, radiation, cigarette smoke, and herbicides can also generate free radicals.

Our defensive line, including our immune system and antioxidants produced by the liver (such as glutathione and superoxide dismutase), needs fuel from outside sources to conquer our health-robbing adversary. Quite simply, the fuel is food, and good dietary decisions tip the odds in a victory against free radical damage.

The Dangers of Oxidized LDL Cholesterol

Much like the rusting of metal on a car, oxidation of LDL cholesterol plays a role in heart disease. The oxidized, low-density lipoprotein cholesterol builds up in the arteries and increases the risk of heart disease, the leading cause of premature death among people with diabetes. Like players on a team, each antioxidant plays a special role in protecting cells and organs from oxidative damage. Therefore, it's important to include all the players in your diet to win the game against diabetes. Let's take a look at some of the superstars you should have on your starting lineup.

The Antioxidant Superstars

With the dedication of researchers and evolution of technology, we are able to measure the levels of antioxidants in specific foods helping us to identify the star players to include in our diet. Remember, digestion, absorption, and methods of cooking play roles in the amount of antioxidants in foods, so be sure to change it up and keep your diet varied. Table 4.1 summarizes the top twenty food sources of antioxidants. You'll find out about the phytonutrients responsible for these free radical–fighting actions in the next section.

TABLE 4.1 Top Twenty Food Sources of Antioxidants

Rank	Food	Serving Size	Total Antioxidant Capacity per Serving
1	Small red beans (dried)	½ cup	13,727
2	Wild blueberries	1 cup	13,427
3	Red kidney beans (dried)	½ cup	13,259
4	Pinto beans	½ cup	11,864
5	Blueberries (cultivated)	1 cup	9,019
6	Cranberries	1 cup (whole)	8,983
7	Artichokes (cooked)	1 cup (hearts)	7,904
8	Blackberries	1 cup	7,701
9	Dried prunes	½ cup	7,291
10	Raspberries	1 cup	6,058
11	Strawberries	1 cup	5,938
12	Red Delicious apples	One	5,900
13	Granny Smith apples	One	5,381
14	Pecans	1 ounce	5,095
15	Sweet cherries	1 cup	4,873
16	Black plums	One	4,844
17	Russet potatoes (cooked)	One	4,649
18	Black beans (dried)	½ cup	4,181
19	Plums	One	4,118
20	Gala apples	One	3,903

Kitchen Prescription

Many factors affect the levels of antioxidants in foods, including the method of cooking. Some antioxidants, such as vitamin C, are water-soluble, while others, such as lycopene and other carotenoids, are lipid- or fat-soluble. In general, lipid-soluble antioxidants are best absorbed by the body when cooked and consumed with a bit of fat (oil), whereas water-soluble foods are best fresh, as cooking destroys these compounds or they are lost in the water. For example, cook your carrots with a little olive oil to maximize the absorption of lipid-soluble carotenoids and gently steam broccoli (instead of boiling) to keep those water-soluble nutrients in the stalks and not left behind in the pot!

Phytonutrient Fuel: A Clean Pass

Much of the good press antioxidants get is due to tiny compounds called *phytonutrients* found inside the fruits, vegetables, legumes, and grains we eat. These phytonutrients (*phyto* meaning plant) protect plants against harsh weather conditions and hungry insects and even heal the wounds made by nibbling moths. With their own defensive lineup, plant foods stand ready to guard against hungry predators trying to take a bite or fungi that hang around trying to drain its resources.

This plant-protection system—essentially antioxidants and phytonutrients—not only serves as defense, but is also to credit for the vibrant colors and delicious flavors of our food. Interestingly, distinguishing colors is a trait common only to humans and a few species of primates. So the foods most appealing to our eyes are also most appealing to our body to prevent and treat diseases.

It should come as no surprise that fruits and vegetables with higher levels of antioxidants produce fresher foods for longer periods of time (shelf life) with less risk of mold. These foods are better equipped to preserve and protect themselves, and when we take a bite, we become the proverbial receiver of those antioxidants and phytonutrients—passing heart-helping nutrients on to us.

Unfortunately, the development of agriculture some ten thousand years ago caused a shift away from our diverse plant-based diet that provided a spectrum of essential vitamins and minerals and tens of thousands of protective phytonutrients. Replacing this delicious and defensive diet with processed foods, refined grains, added oils, sugar, and salt has led to the rise of chronic diseases including heart disease. In fact, today most Americans eat only between two and three servings of fruits and vegetables per day (when the optimum is seven to nine servings), and a minority eat none at all.

Advances in technology have allowed us to further explore compounds in foods on a molecular level, distinguishing among the thousands of plant nutrients in individual foods and food families. This "new nutritional frontier" provides us with critical information on how best we can use foods to reduce cholesterol and protect the heart. It is estimated that twenty-five thousand individual phytonutrients have been identified in fruits, vegetables, and grains, but a large percentage still remain unknown and need to be identified before we can fully understand their health benefits.

Your body's "multiplayer" defense system is assisted by the phytonutrient fuel you feed it. Each time you eat fruits, vegetables, or other antioxidant-rich foods, you catch the pass, and a flood of heart-protecting nutrients enters your bloodstream. Let's take a look at the lineup.

The Vitamins and Minerals That Protect Your Heart

Although we have known about the actions of vitamins and minerals for some time, it is only recently that we have begun to understand their individual roles in heart disease. We offer information on the vitamins and minerals as a percentage of the daily value (DV). Talk with your nutritionist to meet your personal nutrition needs.

Calcium

Calcium is an intracellular messenger and plays a role in mediating the constriction and relaxation of blood vessels, nerve impulse transmission, muscle contraction, and the secretion of hormones including insulin. This common mineral has beneficial effects on lipids and may aid in weight control as well. By forming insoluble soaps with fatty acids in the intestine, calcium helps to prevent the absorption of part of the dietary fat, reducing cholesterol. Talk with your nutritionist to determine if supplementing your diet with calcium, in addition to eating calcium-rich foods, may be appropriate.

 Healing Tip

Cut the Cholesterol. Get calcium in low-fat yogurt (415 mg or 42 percent DV), skim milk (402 mg or 30 percent DV), tofu (204 mg or 20 percent DV), orange juice (200 mg or 20 percent DV), salmon (181 mg or 18 percent DV), kale (94 mg or 9 percent DV), and bok choy (74 mg or 7 percent DV).

Calculating Calcium. The following foods provide the same amount of calcium: 8 ounces of milk = 1 cup of yogurt = 1½ ounces of cheddar cheese = 1½ cups of cooked kale = 2¼ cups of cooked broccoli = 8 cups of cooked spinach.

Eat a variety of calcium-rich foods to maximize your absorption of this important mineral. Visit The Office of Dietary Supplements at http://ods.od.nih.gov/factsheets/calcium.asp to learn more about calcium requirements for men and women at different life stages.

Folate

Folate gets its name from the latin word *folium*, for leaf, and hence is present in good amounts in leafy greens. Folate works in conjunction with vitamin B₆ and vitamin B₁₂ to help recycle homocysteine into methionine. A number of studies have shown that high levels of homocysteine are associated with an increased risk of heart disease.

 Healing Tip

Beans and Greens! If you frequently dine on "beans and greens" you're fine with folate. You can get it in black-eyed peas (105 mcg or 25 percent DV), cooked spinach (100 mcg or 25 percent DV), great northern beans (90 mcg or 20 percent DV), asparagus (85 mcg or 20 percent DV), wheat germ (40 mcg or 10 percent DV), orange juice (35 mcg or 10 percent DV), peas (50 mcg or 15 percent DV), cooked broccoli (45 mcg or 15 percent DV), avocado (45 mcg or 10 percent DV), and peanuts (40 mcg or 10 percent DV).

Magnesium

Magnesium is a mineral involved with blood pressure regulation, insulin function, and heart disease. Some studies have shown that people with higher blood levels of magnesium have a lower risk of heart disease and stroke. Low levels of magnesium increase the risk of abnormal heart rhythms, which may increase the risk of complications after a heart attack.

Healing Tip

Magnificent Magnesium! Get it in halibut (90 mg or 20 percent DV), almonds (80 mg or 20 percent DV), cashews (75 mg or 20 percent DV), soybeans (75 mg or 20 percent DV), spinach (75 mg or 20 percent DV), oatmeal (55 mg or 15 percent DV), potatoes (50 mg or 15 percent DV), peanuts (50 mg or 15 percent DV), black-eyed peas (45 mg or 10 percent DV), yogurt (45 mg or 10 percent DV), baked beans (40 mg or 10 percent DV), and brown rice (40 mg or 10 percent DV).

Vitamins B$_6$ and B$_{12}$

Vitamin B$_{12}$, also called cobalamin, helps maintain healthy nerve cells and red blood cells and is also needed to make DNA. Vitamin B$_{12}$, in conjunction with vitamin B$_6$ and folate, helps to reduce levels of heart-harming homocysteine, a sulfur-containing amino acid. The results of more than eighty studies indicate that even moderately elevated levels of homocysteine in the blood increase the risk of cardiovascular diseases. If you are a vegetarian, speak with your doctor or dietitian about supplementing vitamin B$_{12}$, which is obtained primarily from animal sources.

Healing Tip

Boost Your Bs! Get heart-helping vitamin B_6 in potatoes (0.7 mg or 35 percent DV), garbanzo beans (0.57 mg or 30 percent DV), chicken breast (0.52 mg or 25 percent DV), oatmeal (0.42 mg or 20 percent DV), sunflower seeds (0.23 mg or 10 percent DV), avocado (0.20 mg or 10 percent DV), and cooked spinach (0.14 mg or 8 percent DV). You'll find Vitamin B_{12} in clams (84.1 mcg or 1,400 percent DV), trout (5.4 mcg or 90 percent DV), salmon (4.9 mcg or 80 percent DV), yogurt (1.4 mcg or 25 percent DV), tuna (1 mcg or 15 percent DV), and milk (0.9 mcg or 15 percent DV).

Vitamin C

Vitamin C is a water-soluble antioxidant also known as ascorbic acid. Antioxidant nutrients, as we discussed earlier in the chapter, have important roles in reducing free radical damage associated with cardiovascular disease as well as many other chronic diseases including diabetes, macular degeneration, cataracts, asthma, and cancer.

Healing Tip

Orange You Healthy? Get your daily dose of vitamin C in medium oranges (78 mg or 104 percent DV), medium grapefruit (132 mg or 178 percent DV), blueberries (14 mg or 19 percent DV), strawberries (122 mg or 163 percent DV), mangoes (57 mg or 76 percent DV), papaya (94 mg or 125 percent DV), cantaloupe (70 mg or 93 percent DV), watermelon (12 mg or 16 percent DV), sweet potatoes (18 mg or 24 percent DV), green peppers (95 mg or 125 percent DV), and red peppers (226 mg or 301 percent DV).

Vitamin E

Vitamin E is a fat-soluble vitamin that exists in eight different forms, each with its own specific function in the body. *Alphatocopherol* is the name of the most active form of vitamin E in humans and is a powerful antioxidant. Researchers have found that oxidative changes to LDL cholesterol promote blockages in coronary arteries that may lead to heart attacks. Vitamin E may help to prevent or delay coronary heart disease by limiting the oxidation of LDL cholesterol, and it may help prevent the formation of blood clots, which could lead to a heart attack. A study of approximately ninety thousand nurses suggested that the incidence of heart disease was 30 percent to 40 percent lower among nurses with the highest intake of vitamin E from diet and supplements. While vitamin E from foods in the diet (such as those listed in the following) may have beneficial effects on the heart, the evidence for supplements is still inconclusive.

 Healing Tip

Es to Please! Vitamin E is found in wheat germ oil (20.3 mg or 100 percent DV), almonds (7.4 mg or 40 percent DV), sunflower seeds (6 mg or 40 percent DV), hazelnuts (4.3 mg or 20 percent DV), peanuts (2.2 mg or 10 percent DV), mango (0.9 mg or 6 percent DV), broccoli (1.2 mg or 6 percent DV), spinach (1.6 mg or 6 percent DV), and kiwi (1.1 mg or 6 percent DV).

The Phytonutrients That Protect Your Heart

Don't let the big names of these tiny compounds scare you. They deliver a powerful cholesterol-cutting punch even when you don't call them by name. The important thing is to include the full spectrum every day to keep your heart healthy.

Phenolic Phytonutrients and Flavonoids

Phenolics represent a very large category of more than two thousand phytonutrients. The term *phenol* comes from the chemical structure of these phytonutrients that varies from having one to several "phenol groups." These powerful phenol groups have the ability to sweep up many free radicals as they circulate through the bloodstream, reducing damage to cells and oxidation of LDL cholesterol. Considered to be some of the most powerful antioxidants, phenolics are being studied for their ability to slow the aging process and also have anti-inflammatory, clot-busting, and heart-protective effects.

Flavonoids are molecular compounds that serve as a defense mechanism; they are found only in plants. Because plants don't have the fight-or-flight option of animals, they must protect themselves chemically, and flavonoids make the plant tissue unappetizing to fungi, insects, and other organisms harmful to plants. Every plant makes flavonoids, but they tend to be concentrated in the leaves and fruit. For that reason, fruits tend to be a richer source of flavonoids than many vegetables.

The Women's Health Study surveyed nearly forty thousand women to determine the association between flavonoids in the diet and the risk of heart disease. Women eating the most flavonoid-rich foods had a 35 percent reduction in cardiovascular events. Let's take a look at the specific flavonoids in foods and how each member allies forces to help your heart.

 Healing Tip

Fabulous flavonoids can be found in apples, broccoli, celery, citrus fruits, cocoa, eggplant, endive, grapes, grapefruit, leeks, onion, parsley, raspberries, red wine, strawberries, and tea.

Tannins. These substances, primarily found in tea, have been studied for their actions on inflammation and their ability to thin the blood. Intake of five flavonoids—the majority of which were derived from tea consumption—was found to be inversely associated with dying from cardiovascular disease.

Healing Tip

Drink to Your Health! Get tannins in green tea, oolong tea, black tea, sorghum, red wine, and coffee.

Anthocyanins. These brightly colored compounds have recently been found to stop the oxidation and reduce levels of LDL cholesterol. They were also found to reduce the stickiness of platelets in the blood that can form a dangerous clot. They have beneficial effects on fat cells (adipocytes) and reduce inflammatory compounds called cytokines.

Kitchen Prescription

Berry Delicious Medicine! You can find these compounds most readily in red-blue fruits including blueberries, raspberries, lingonberries, cherries, currants, pomegranates, strawberries, Concord grapes, cranberries, and elderberries. Buy them frozen, and add to smoothies or thaw for a quick addition to cereal.

Beta-Glucan. As soluble fiber, beta-glucan, found in high concentrations in oats and barley, helps to reduce cholesterol. In fact, men and women consuming 5.8 grams of beta-glucan for four weeks saw a 10 percent reduction in their LDL cholesterol in a recent study. In 1997, the FDA approved a health claim on food products that "a diet high in soluble fiber from whole oats and low in saturated fat and cholesterol may reduce the risk of heart disease." The FDA concluded that at least 3 grams of beta-glucan from oats should be consumed to achieve a reduction in cholesterol.

 Kitchen Prescription

Old-Fashioned Remedy. Try our recipe for Cinnamon Raisin Scones in Chapter 9 for a delicious way to get your cholesterol-cutting beta-glucan.

Sterols and Stanols. Found naturally in vegetable oils, nuts, cereals, and beans, as well as in the new cholesterol-lowering dairy spread, sterols and stanols help to reduce LDL cholesterol levels by decreasing its absorption in the intestine. A variety of these compounds exist, with names like campesterol, sitosterol, and stigmasterol. An analysis of fourteen studies concluded that getting 2 grams of stanols or sterols reduced LDL cholesterol by 9 to 14 percent.

 Healing Tip

Look for nonhydrogenated sterol margarine spreads in the dairy section, such as Take Control and Benecol, to help cut your cholesterol, but make sure you're eating lots of carotenoid-rich fruits and vegetables (discussed later in this chapter). Sterols and stanols reduce these heart-helping nutrients.

Catechins. These substances are most often found in black, green, and oolong tea, as well as in red wine. A 2005 study published in the *Journal of Nutritional Biochemistry* gave two cups of green tea (containing 250 mg of catechins) to healthy participants for forty-two days. Compared with the participants in the study not drinking tea, the tea drinkers enjoyed an increase in antioxidants in the blood and a significant reduction in LDL cholesterol.

 Kitchen Prescription

Cholesterol-Cutting Catechins! An average cup of brewed green or black tea has 150 to 200 milligrams of flavonoids—including catechins. Steep your green tea for two minutes to maximize the antioxidant benefits.

Quercetin. This naturally occurring antioxidant helps to reduce the body's absorption of cholesterol and encourage its removal from the body. A 2005 animal study published in *Free Radical Resolution* examined the effects of quercetin on a high-cholesterol diet. The subjects on a high-cholesterol diet who also received quercetin saw a decrease in total cholesterol, triglycerides, and fatty acids in the blood and vessels of the heart.

 Healing Tip

Don't Quit the Quercetin! You can get it in red grapes, red and yellow onions, broccoli, and apples.

Isoflavones. Isoflavones are *phytoestrogens* (plant estrogens) that may help to reduce cholesterol. Numerous isoflavones exist in plants such as soybeans, including diadzein, genistein, and glycitein. The FDA says that 25 grams of soy protein as part of a diet low in saturated fat and cholesterol may reduce the risk of heart disease. Studies show that soy, because of isoflavones such as genistein, may be useful in preventing heart disease and improving cholesterol levels.

 Healing Tip

Oh Soy! Get a daily dose of isoflavones in soy products such as tofu, soy milk, tempeh, and edamame. The isoflavone content varies widely among soybean varieties and from product to product based on manufacturing process and source of soy protein; read labels to determine the approximate isoflavone content of foods.

 Culinary caution: Talk with your doctor if you have any type of cancer and choose isoflavones from whole foods as opposed to supplements and isolated isoflavone products.

Resveratrol. A substance found in the skins of red and white grapes (as well as peanuts), this phytonutrient helps to reduce triglycerides and LDL cholesterol levels. It also helps prevent the unnecessary blood clots that can trigger serious problems such as heart attack or stroke.

 Healing Tip

Resveratrol is found in red wine and red grape juice. It is not found in white wine because the grape skins, which contain the resveratrol, are discarded early in the manufacturing process.

Curcumin. Credited for the unique flavors and golden color of curries, curcumin is a potent antioxidant that adds heart healthy flavor.

Kitchen Prescription

Spicy Protection! Curcumin is found in turmeric, and you can get the benefits of this amazing phytonutrient with our recipe for Indian Spice Mix.

Indian Spice Mix
2 teaspoons ground turmeric
8 teaspoons dry mustard
4 teaspoons ground fenugreek
4 teaspoons ground cumin
2 teaspoons ground ginger
2 teaspoons ground coriander
2 teaspoons ground cloves
½ teaspoon ground cinnamon

Combine all ingredients in a small bowl with an airtight lid. Shake well to blend. Store in a cool, dry place, sealed. Add to chicken, fish, and bean dishes.

Makes about 24½ teaspoons

Gingerols. These aromatic phytonutrients are found in—what else?—ginger. This compound, along with others in the ginger family, have been found to prevent the oxidation of LDL cholesterol. Ginger is a member of the Zingiberaceae family, which also includes turmeric.

Kitchen Prescription

Try ginger in our Shanghai Chicken Kabobs in Chapter 9.

Citrus Flavonoids. Citrus foods provide an abundance of heart-healthy flavonoids such as hesperidin, naringin, and nobiletin. Let's take a look at the health a-peel of each.

Hesperidin, found in oranges, might help to reduce total cholesterol as well as triglycerides.

Naringin, found in high concentrations in grapefruits, helps to reduce LDL cholesterol and boost HDL. A 2004 study published in *Clinical Nutrition* compared the cholesterol-lowering effects of naringin with the cholesterol-reducing drug lovastatin. After eight weeks, both the naringin and lovastatin significantly reduced total and LDL cholesterol levels, while increasing HDL cholesterol.

Nobiletin, found primarily in tangerines, was reported in 2005 in the journal *Atherosclerosis* to reduce cholesterol and help to protect the arteries.

 Kitchen Prescription

Put the Squeeze on Heart Disease! Get a heart-healthy dose of these cholesterol-cutting citrus flavonoids in our Carotene Cooler in Chapter 9.

Carotenoid Phytonutrients

Carotenoids, a group of more than six hundred related nutrients, have received substantial attention both because of their pro-vitamin and antioxidant roles. In 2003, the *American Journal of Clinical Nutrition* reported results from the Nurses' Health Study on carotenoids and heart disease risk in women. The study followed 73,286 female nurses for twelve years and found the women eating more alpha-carotene- or beta-carotene-rich foods enjoyed a lower risk of heart disease. Carotenoids have also been found to reduce the risk of stroke. Researchers agree that getting the spectrum of carotenoids is the best strategy to improve your health and get their maximum antioxidant benefits.

One of the side effects of eating *phytosterols* (the margarine spreads available in the dairy section) to reduce cholesterol levels is that they also reduce levels of carotenoids in the body, making it especially important to get lots of carotenoid-rich fruits and vegetables.

It is also important to mention that taking carotenoid supplements can pose health threats, including increasing the risk of death for those who smoke. The best way to get your carotenoids is through the foods we'll discuss here, ensuring your body gets the full spectrum of disease-fighting phytonutrients.

 Kitchen Prescription

Fourteen-Carrot Protection! As fat-soluble compounds, you can get the most protection by cooking these foods and adding a little oil. It helps make the phytonutrients more available to your body so more gets into your bloodstream to protect the heart.

Lycopene is well known for its ability to protect the heart by reducing the oxidation of LDL cholesterol. The Kuopio Ischemic Heart Disease (KIHD) Risk Factor Study found that men with the lowest levels of lycopene had a threefold increase in risk for a heart attack or stroke.

 Kitchen Prescription

Love Your Lycopene! Other than tomatoes, you can get lycopene in watermelon, guava, papaya, apricots, pink grapefruit, and blood oranges. It's fat-soluble too, so cook those tomatoes well, add some extra-virgin olive oil, and toss with your favorite pasta!

Lutein and *zeaxanthin* are most famous for their role in reducing the risk of age-related macular degeneration, and emerging evidence suggests these yellow-green compounds may also aid in preventing heart disease and stroke.

 Healing Tip

Outta Sight! Get lutein and zeaxanthin in broccoli, kale, spinach, and egg yolks.

Allylic Sulfur Compounds

Derived mainly from the allium, or onion, family, these phytonutrients give the characteristic bite to onions, garlic, and other relatives of this bulb group. These compounds have been found to protect the heart, thin the blood, and help reduce cholesterol.

Ajoene is found in garlic and is known for its blood-thinning and cholesterol-lowering properties.

Allicin is formed in garlic when an intact clove of garlic is crushed. An odorless amino acid, alliin, is enzymatically converted by allinase into allicin when the cloves are crushed. Allicin is thought to be one of the most biologically active compounds in garlic, reducing the oxidation of LDL cholesterol.

Sulfides are also found in garlic as well as in cabbage, broccoli, brussels sprouts, and other members of the crucifer family. *Diallyl disulfide (DADS)*, a substance that is formed from the compounds present in garlic, is known to increase levels of detoxifying enzymes in the body, including glutathione. Sulfides act as antithrombotic compounds (clot busters) and may protect against heart disease and strokes by thinning the blood, preventing oxidation of LDL cholesterol, and reducing blood pressure.

Kitchen Prescription

Cloves of Protection! Don't let anyone tell you garlic breath isn't beautiful. Crush garlic and mix in with a simple dressing of extra-virgin olive oil and balsamic vinegar and drizzle over a big mixed green salad full of phytonutrients, or enjoy it in our recipe here for Garlicky Bruschetta.

Garlicky Bruschetta
4 tomatoes, chopped
4 garlic cloves, crushed
½ shallot, diced
½ cup chopped fresh basil
¼ cup extra-virgin olive oil
8 slices whole-grain Italian bread

Mix all cholesterol-lowering ingredients together (except bread). Let stand for ten minutes. Toast whole-grain bread and top with tomato mixture for a dose of ajoene, allicin, sulfides, and lycopene.

Serves 8 (serving size: 1 slice bread with ¼ cup tomato mixture)

Now that you have learned about how certain foods that contain fats, carbs, antioxidants, and phytonutrients can help you to reduce cholesterol and protect against heart disease, you can read the next chapter to find a whole list of foods to incorporate all of these elements into your daily diet for optimum health.

Cholesterol-Lowering Foods

EACH FRUIT, VEGETABLE, legume, or grain—like a team player or a note in a symphony—adds a nutritional element valuable to cutting your cholesterol and preventing heart disease. Some people are under the dangerous misconception that the cost of an unhealthy diet can be offset by taking nutritional supplements. *Wrong!* Because many phytonutrients have yet to be identified, and because other elements—such as fiber, healthy fats, and the like—aren't in those pills, we're fighting the battle against heart disease with the wrong weapons. Now that you've learned about the spectrum of cholesterol-reducing nutrients, fats, and carbohydrates, let's look at the individual foods that work together to help reduce your cholesterol and stave off heart disease.

The Synergy of Foods

With the diligent work of scientists worldwide and the evolution of technology, we have isolated and identified approximately twenty-five thousand unique phytonutrients in hundreds of different types of plant foods. Through research, we're learning that by combining these foods, the bioactive compounds work together, or synergistically, to increase health benefits. For example, when oranges, apples, grapes, and blueberries were tested both alone and together, the antioxidant activity was five times higher for the combined fruit salad than for the individual fruits.

Although particular groups of fruits and vegetables have been found to be especially protective for reducing cholesterol, research has pointed to the conclusion that lowering your cholesterol and preventing heart disease is best achieved by food synergy. Now let's explore the families of foods and their unique heart-protective properties (seen in Table 5.1).

TABLE 5.1 Foods and Their Heart-Helping Properties

Group/Family	Foods	Phytochemicals
Cruciferae (crucifer family)	Broccoli, brussels sprouts, cabbage, cauliflower, collard greens, kale, kohlrabi, mustard greens, radishes, rutabaga, turnips, watercress	Isothiocyanates, indoles, nitriles, sulforaphane, chlorophyll
Cucurbitaceae (the melon and squash family)	Cantaloupes, cucumbers, honeydew melons, summer squash (pumpkin, zucchini), winter squash (acorn, butternut)	Carotenoids, beta-carotene, alpha-carotene, beta-cryptoxanthin, zeaxanthin, lutein
Labitae (mint family)	Basil, mint, oregano, rosemary, sage, thyme	Terpenoids, menthol, chlorophyll
Leguminosae (bean family)	Alfalfa sprouts, beans, peas, soybeans	Phytoestrogens, lignans, protease inhibitors, isoflavones, saponins

TABLE 5.1 *(continued)*

Group/Family	Foods	Phytochemicals
Liliaceae (lily family)	Asparagus, chives, garlic, leeks, onions, shallots	Sulfur compounds, sulfides, allicin, diallyl sulfide
Rutacea (citrus family)	*Grapefruit, lemons, limes, oranges, tangerines	Limonene, carotenoids, lycopene (blood oranges and pink grapefruits), vitamin C, hesperidin, naringin, nobiletin
Solanaceae (solanum/ nightshade family	Eggplant, peppers, potatoes, tomatoes	Lycopene, carotenoids, terpenes
Umbelliferae (umbel family)	Anise, caraway, carrots, celeriac, celery, chervil, cilantro, coriander, cumin, dill, fennel, parsley, parsnips	Carotenoids, beta-carotene, alpha carotene, beta-cryptoxanthin, zeaxanthin, lutein, chlorophyll
Zingiberaceae (ginger family)	Ginger, turmeric	Curcumin, gingerols, zingibain
Tea family	Black tea, green tea, oolong tea, white tea varieties	Catechins, tannins, polyphenols, epigallo-catechin gallate (EGCG), theaflavins

*Check with your doctor before eating grapefruit, as it can have interactions with different medications, especially statins.

Color-Coded Cuisine

Use your plate like a canvas and paint to your heart's content! David Heber, Ph.D., of the UCLA Center for Human Nutrition in Los Angeles, introduced a concept that groups foods by color to simplify eating for optimum health and disease prevention. It is not necessary to know the names of the thousands of phytonutrients present in foods to reap their health benefits. In fact, choosing a variety of foods from all of the families we have described offers the complete spectrum of nutrients needed to protect us from disease. The same phytonutrients that keep our cells healthy also give fruits and vegetables their colors and indicate their unique physiological roles. By color-coding our cuisine, we can translate the science of phytonutrient nutrition into delicious dishes. Let's take a look at what the colors mean.

❖ **Blue and purple.** Blue and purple fruits and vegetables contain varying amounts of health-promoting phytonutrients such as anthocyanins and phenolics. Anthocyanins are currently being studied for their ability to stop the oxidation of LDL cholesterol and their ability to reduce inflammatory compounds.

❖ **Green.** Green vegetables contain varying amounts of phytonutrients such as lutein and indoles, which interest researchers because of their potential antioxidant, health-promoting benefits. They are also full of folate—an important B vitamin that helps to reduce levels of heart-harming homocysteine.

❖ **White.** White, tan, and brown fruits and vegetables contain varying amounts of phytonutrients of interest to scientists. These include sulfides and allicin, found in the garlic and onion family, which help protect the heart by reducing the oxidation of LDL cholesterol.

❖ **Yellow and orange.** Yellow and orange fruits and vegetables contain varying amounts of antioxidants such as vitamin C as well as carotenoids and flavonoids. Citrus fruits have several unique flavonoids in their cholesterol-cutting arsenal including nobiletin, naringin, and hesperidin.

❖ **Red.** Specific phytonutrients in the red group that are being studied for their health-promoting properties include lycopene and anthocyanins. Lycopene, a powerful antioxidant found in the highest concentrations in cooked tomato products, is particularly protective of the heart.

A to Z Foods: Your Cholesterol-Lowering Team

Cut your cholesterol deliciously! In this section, we take the colors one step further and discover the individual foods in the cholesterol-lowering team. We'll also show you what to look for when selecting, tell you how to store for optimum flavor and nutritional benefits, and suggest some recipes from Chapter 9 that incorporate these foods. We have included the nutrients in foods as a percentage of the RDA, or recommended daily allowance. To learn more about how these individual nutrients promote health and protect your heart, refer back to Chapter 4. Please note that the list in this book is limited; visit our website, healinggourmet.com, for more information.

 Healing Tip

Look for locally grown, organic produce that has been grown without the use of chemical pesticides. Also, try organic dairy products, free-range poultry, and wild fish to reduce your consumption of chemicals and hormones.

Apples

Grown in temperate zones throughout the world and cultivated for at least three thousand years, apple varieties now number well into the thousands. The apple has been called the "king of fruits," and for good reason. Apples contain a soluble fiber called pectin, which reduces total cholesterol and LDL without affecting the beneficial HDL levels. They also contain flavonoids that help to protect the heart by halting the oxidation of LDL cholesterol.

❖ **Serving.** One apple (5 oz) with skin contains 81 calories, 0.3 gram protein, 22 grams carbohydrates, no fat, no cholesterol, and 5 grams dietary fiber. The same serving provides 13 percent of the RDA for vitamin C (4.8 mg) and 8 percent of the RDA for vitamin E (0.8 mg). Apples also contain phenols, chlorogenic acid, pectin, quercetin, flavonoids, boron, and salicylates.

❖ **Selecting and storing.** Available year-round, apples' peak season is from September through November when newly harvested. Buy firm, well-colored apples with a fresh (never musty) fragrance. The skins should be smooth and free of bruises and gouges. Store apples in a cool, dark place. They do well placed in a plastic bag and stored in the refrigerator.

 Kitchen Prescription

Try our Apple and Cranberry Crisp for a delicious breakfast or dessert snack that's packed with flavonoids and heart-helping fiber.

Artichokes

Vegetable flowers that are picked and eaten before they turn into a "real" flower, artichokes are a European staple with more than forty varieties in existence. The compounds known as luteolin and cynaroside found in artichokes stop the creation (biosynthesis) of cholesterol in the liver, helping to reduce cholesterol.

❖ **Serving.** One artichoke, boiled (4.2 oz), contains 60 calories, 4.2 grams protein, 13.4 grams carbohydrates, 0.2 gram fat, no cholesterol, and 6.5 grams dietary fiber. The same serving provides 15 percent of the RDA for folate (61.2 mcg), 16 percent of the RDA for vitamin C (12 mg), 12 percent of the RDA for magnesium (47 mg), 11 percent of the RDA for iron (1.6 mg), and 425 milligrams potassium. Artichokes also contain cynaroside, luteolin, dicaffeoylquinic, and dicaffeoyltartaric acids.

❖ **Selecting and storing.** Globe artichokes are available year-round, with the peak season from March through May. Buy deep green, heavy-for-their-size artichokes with a tight leaf formation. The leaves should "squeak" when pressed together. Heavy browning on an artichoke usually indicates it's beyond its prime. Store unwashed artichokes in a plastic bag in the refrigerator for up to four days; wash just before cooking. Artichoke hearts are available frozen and canned; artichoke bottoms are available canned.

 Kitchen Prescription

Try our Black Bean Salad with Artichokes, Pepper, and Goat Cheese to get these great globes on your plate. Also, look for canned artichoke hearts in water in the supermarket to add to your favorite pasta, chicken, and fish dishes.

Asparagus

A member of the lily family, the edible part of asparagus is actually the young underground sprout or shoot. A serving of these spears provides 48 percent of the RDA for folate, a vitamin that helps to reduce heart-harming homocysteine. More than eighty studies show that even moderately elevated levels of homocysteine in the blood increase the risk of heart disease.

❖ **Serving.** One-half cup of raw asparagus contains 15 calories, 1.5 grams protein, 2.5 grams carbohydrates, 0.1 gram fat, no cholesterol, and 1.3 grams dietary fiber. The same serving provides 6 percent of the RDA for vitamin A (60 RE), 48 percent of the RDA for folate (95 mcg), 37 percent of the RDA for vitamin C (22.1 mg), 5 percent of the RDA for vitamin B$_6$ (0.1 mg), 3 percent of the RDA for iron (0.4 mg), and 218 milligrams potassium.

❖ **Selecting and storing.** The optimum season for fresh asparagus lasts from February through June, although hothouse asparagus is available year-round in some regions. It's best cooked the same day it's purchased but will keep, tightly wrapped in a plastic bag, three to four days in the refrigerator. Or, store standing upright in about an inch of water, covering the container with a plastic bag.

 Kitchen Prescription

Spear-ited Health! Before cooking your asparagus, fill a glass with spring water and two crushed garlic cloves. Cut the base of your asparagus spears, place them in the glass, and let it stand twenty minutes. The spears will take up the water, making them crisper, and the garlic will add flavor and additional phytonutrients.

Avocados

Native to the tropics and subtropics, avocados are a unique fruit and concentrated source of nutrients. The California avocado has a smooth skin, while the Florida avocado ("alligator pear") has a tough and wrinkled exterior. More like a nut than a fruit, these South American natives supply heart-healthy monounsaturated fat, folate, vitamin B_6, and magnesium to reduce cholesterol and levels of heart-harming homocysteine. Holy guacamole!

❖ **Serving.** One (6 oz) avocado contains 204 calories, 3.8 grams protein, 13.3 grams carbohydrates, 17 grams fat, no cholesterol, and 9.3 grams dietary fiber. The same serving provides 19 percent of the RDA for vitamin A (186 RE), 15 percent of the RDA for folate (60 mcg), 40 percent of the RDA for vitamin C (24 mg), 8 percent of the RDA for vitamin B_6 (0.13 mg), 30 percent of the RDA for niacin (5.9 mg), 27 percent of the RDA for thiamin (0.4 mg), 26 percent of the RDA for magnesium (104 mg), 22 percent of the RDA for riboflavin (0.4 mg), 11 percent of the RDA for iron (1.6 mg), and 1,484 milligrams potassium.

❖ **Selecting and storing.** Like many fruits, avocados ripen best off the tree. Ripe avocados yield to gentle palm pressure, but firm, unripe avocados are what are usually found in the market. Select those that are unblemished and heavy for their size. To speed the ripening process, place several avocados in a paper bag and set aside at room temperature for two to four days. Ripe avocados can be stored in the refrigerator several days. Once avocado flesh is cut and exposed to the air, it tends to discolor rapidly; adding lemon or lime juice helps to prevent discoloration.

Kitchen Prescription

Awesome avocados make the creamy dressing for our Wild Rice Salad. They're also perfect right off the tree, pitted, with a squeeze of lemon and your favorite mixed greens.

Barley

Beige and shaped like a flattened oval, this grain is usually sold pearled, where it is hulled and polished to cook more quickly. Barley can also be found in quick-cooking, whole hulled, Job's tears (large hulled grains), grits flakes, and flour varieties. Hulled, also called *whole-grain*, barley has only the outer husk removed and is the most nutritious form of the grain. Scotch barley is husked and coarsely ground. Barley grits are hulled barley grains that have been cracked into medium-coarse pieces. Used to make beer, whiskey, and cattle feed, barley is a gluten grain that should be avoided by those with gluten sensitivity. Barley provides heart-healthy tocotrienols (a form of vitamin E), which help to reduce the oxidation of low-density lipoprotein and reduce overall cholesterol levels.

❖ **Serving.** One-half cup of cooked pearled barley contains 97 calories, 1.8 grams protein, 22.3 grams carbohydrates, 0.4 gram fat, no cholesterol, and 4.4 grams dietary fiber. The same serving provides 6 percent of the RDA for folate (12.6 mcg), 8 percent of the RDA for niacin (1.6 mg), and 7 percent of the RDA for iron (1.1 mg).

❖ **Selecting and storing.** Hulled and Scotch barley and barley grits are generally found in health food stores. Pearl barley has also had the bran removed and has been steamed and polished. It comes in three sizes—coarse, medium, and fine—and is good in soups and stews. Store in an airtight container in a cool, dry place.

 Healing Tip

Opt for hulled barley that still has its germ and bran layers intact, which delivers cholesterol-mopping fiber to protect the heart.

Beans

Beans, part of the legume family, are a good protein source and a low-glycemic-index food. They provide a bevy of phytonutrients to benefit the heart, including phytoestrogens, folate, insoluble fiber, and saponins. Make these packages of protection a mainstay in your diet for optimum health. A national study of more than ten thousand people showed that eating beans, peas, or lentils four times a week cut heart disease by 22 percent. Bean up!

* **Serving.** One-half cup of cooked black beans contains 113 calories, 7.6 grams protein, 20.4 grams carbohydrates, 0.4 gram fat, no cholesterol, and 7.5 grams dietary fiber. The same serving size provides 32 percent of the RDA for folate (64.2 mcg), 13 percent of the RDA for magnesium (51.6 mg), and 270.2 milligrams potassium.

* **Selecting and storing.** Dried beans must usually be soaked in water for several hours or overnight to rehydrate them before cooking. Beans labeled "quick-cooking" have been presoaked and redried before packaging, and they require no presoaking and take considerably less time to prepare. The texture of these "quick" beans, however, is not as firm to the bite as regular dried beans. Store dried beans in an airtight container for up to a year.

 Kitchen Prescription

Try our Black Bean Burritos for a healthy twist on a classic.

Blueberries

These berries have been enjoyed by Native Americans and pilgrims and are among the best-known sources of antioxidants. A true-blue health crusader, blueberries deliver a class of flavonoids called anthocyanins that are potent antioxidants and help reduce the oxidation of LDL cholesterol.

✤ **Serving.** One cup of blueberries contains 82 calories, 1 gram protein, 20.5 grams carbohydrates, 0.6 gram fat, no cholesterol, and 3.5 grams dietary fiber. The same serving provides 315 percent of the RDA for vitamin C (189 mg) and 129 milligrams potassium.

✤ **Selecting and storing.** Choose blueberries that are firm, uniform in size, and indigo blue with a silvery frost. Discard shriveled or moldy berries. Do not wash until ready to use, and store (preferably in a single layer) in a moisture-proof container in the refrigerator for up to five days.

 Kitchen Prescription

You can get these blue gems in our Berry Blast, but that's only one of many ways to enjoy these nutritional powerhouses. Buy them frozen, microwave them, and add them to breakfast cereal for a no-fuss fix full of flavor and phytonutrients.

Broccoli

A descendant of cabbage, broccoli is a member of the cruciferous family of vegetables. Although most broccoli is green, in times past, purple, red, cream, and brown varieties were popular. These trees to ease disease contain a flavonoid called *quercetin* that helps to reduce cholesterol in the blood and protect against heart disease.

✤ **Serving.** One-half cup of cooked broccoli contains 23 calories, 2.3 grams protein, 6 grams carbohydrates, 0.2 gram fat, no cholesterol, and 2.6 grams dietary fiber. The same serving provides 11 percent of the RDA for vitamin A (110 RE), 27 percent of the RDA for folate (53.3 mcg), 82 percent of the RDA for vitamin C (49 mg), 10 percent of the RDA for vitamin B_6 (0.2 mg), 6 percent of the RDA for iron (0.9 mg), and 127 milligrams potassium.

✤ **Selecting and storing.** Look for broccoli with a deep, strong color—green or green with purple. The buds should be tightly closed, and the leaves should be crisp. Refrigerate unwashed, in an airtight bag, for up to four days.

 Kitchen Prescription

Lightly steam broccoli, and add a squeeze of lemon and a shake of Parmesan cheese for the perfect accompaniment to virtually any meal.

Buckwheat

A triangular seed from a fruit relative of rhubarb and sorrel, buckwheat has a nutty flavor and is sold roasted (kasha), whole-grain cracked, in unroasted groats grits, or ground into flour. A good source of sterols and flavonoids, buckwheat has been found in both animal and human studies to help to reduce cholesterol.

✤ **Serving.** One-half cup of cooked buckwheat groats contains 77 calories, 2.8 grams protein, 16.8 grams carbohydrates, 0.5 gram fat, no cholesterol, and 27 grams dietary fiber. The same serving provides 13 percent of the RDA for magnesium (50.5 mg), 7 percent of the RDA for folate (13.9 mcg), and 5 percent of the RDA for iron (0.8 mg).

✤ **Selecting and storing.** Buckwheat groats are the hulled, crushed kernels, which are usually cooked in a manner similar to rice. Groats come in coarse, medium, and fine grinds. Kasha, which is roasted buckwheat groats, has a toastier, more nutty flavor. All can be stored in an airtight container in a cool, dry place.

Healing Tip

Refer back to Chapter 3 to learn about how whole grains, like buckwheat, help to reduce cholesterol, stabilize blood sugar, and stave off heart disease.

Canola Oil

Derived from canola seed, this is minimal in saturated fat. Canola oil provides heart-healthy fats including monounsaturated fat, omega-3 fatty acids, and omega-6 fatty acids.

❖ **Serving.** One tablespoon of canola oil contains 124 calories, no protein, no carbohydrates, 14 grams fat, 1 gram saturated fatty acids, 8 grams monounsaturated fatty acids, 4.2 grams polyunsaturated fatty acids, 1.2 grams omega-3s, no cholesterol, and no dietary fiber. The same serving provides 13 percent of the RDA for vitamin E (2.9 mg).

❖ **Selecting and storing.** Store canola oil in a cool, dry place away from sunlight.

Kitchen Prescription

Canola oil is a light oil perfect for sautéing or using in baked goods. Its neutral flavor makes it a culinary standout for both sweet and savory dishes.

Cantaloupes

These orange-fleshed melons were named after the Italian town of Cantalupa, meaning "wolf howl." They deliver a good dose of vitamin C, along with a powerful punch of carotenoids that may help to reduce the oxidation of LDL cholesterol.

❖ **Serving.** One half raw cantaloupe (9.5 oz) contains 95 calories, 2.5 grams protein, 22.4 grams carbohydrates, 0.8 gram fat, no cholesterol, and 2.5 grams dietary fiber. The same serving provides 86 percent of the RDA for vitamin A (861 RE), 23 percent of the RDA for folate (45.5 mcg), 186 percent of the RDA for vitamin C (112.7 mg), 20 percent of the RDA for vitamin B_6 (0.4 mg), and 825 milligrams potassium.

❖ **Selecting and storing.** Choose cantaloupes that are heavy for their size; have a sweet, fruity fragrance; have a thick, well-raised netting; and yield slightly to pressure at the blossom end. Avoid melons with soft spots or an overly strong odor. Store unripe cantaloupes at room temperature, and keep ripe melons in the refrigerator. Cantaloupes easily absorb other food odors, so if refrigerating for more than a day or two, wrap the melon in plastic wrap.

 Healing Tip

Before cutting into these delicious melons, make sure you wash well as bacteria from the outside gets transferred to the inside with the knife blade.

Carrots

As root vegetables that spread from the Middle East to Greece, Rome, and later Europe, the earliest carrots were not orange but multicolored. In the 1500s, the carrot showed up in Western Europe, and Dutch cross-breeders developed the modern, orange carrot over the following century. Carrots are of course full of carotenoids—those antioxidant compounds that help to protect the heart by stopping the oxidation of LDL cholesterol.

✤ **Serving.** One medium carrot (2.5 oz) contains 31 calories, 0.7 gram protein, 5.6 grams carbohydrates, 0.1 gram fat, no cholesterol, and 2 grams dietary fiber. The same serving also provides 202 percent of the RDA for vitamin A (2,025 RE), 5 percent of the RDA for folate (10 mcg), 11 percent of the RDA for vitamin C (6.7 mg), and 233 milligrams potassium.

✤ **Selecting and storing.** When selecting carrots, choose those that are firm and smooth. Avoid those with cracks or any that have begun to soften and wither. Remove carrot greenery as soon as possible because it robs the roots of moisture and vitamins. Store carrots in a plastic bag in the refrigerator's vegetable bin. Avoid storing them near apples, which emit ethylene gas that can give carrots a bitter taste.

 Kitchen Prescription

Rooted in Health! Try our Carrot Ginger Bisque for a unique twist on this common root veggie. Cooking the carrots makes those fat-soluble phytonutrients more easily absorbed by the body so you get the maximum health benefits. Soup's on!

Cherries

Close cousins to the plum, cherries can be sweet or sour, red or black. Pick cherries for their abundance of flavonoids that help to protect the heart.

❖ **Serving.** Ten sweet, raw cherries (2.4 oz) contain 50 calories, 0.9 gram protein, 11.3 grams carbohydrates, 0.7 gram fat, no cholesterol, and 1.5 grams dietary fiber. The same serving provides 8 percent of the RDA for vitamin C (4.8 mg), 2 percent of the RDA for iron (0.3 mg), and 152 milligrams potassium.

❖ **Selecting and storing.** Most fresh cherries are available from May (June for sour cherries) through August. Choose brightly colored, shiny, plump cherries. Sweet cherries should be firm but not hard, and sour varieties should be medium firm. Store unwashed cherries in a plastic bag in the refrigerator.

 Kitchen Prescription

Not the Pits! Cherries deliver serious benefits to your cardiac muscle. Try them in our Flavonoid Freeze, or buy them frozen, microwave them, and add them to yogurts or breakfast cereals for health on high speed.

Cocoa

Cocoa originated in South America, where it was enjoyed by the Aztecs, Mayans, and other cultures. Introduced by European explorers to the Old World, cocoa became popular when spices, sugar, vanilla, and cinnamon were added to bitter-tasting recipes. Research shows that delicious dark cocoa—a rich source of flavonoids—helps to reduce the oxidation of LDL cholesterol and increases the protective HDL cholesterol.

❖ **Serving.** One cup of hot cocoa (1 tablespoon cocoa with nonfat milk) contains 148 calories, 9.5 grams protein, 30 grams carbohydrates, 9 grams fat, 2 milligrams cholesterol, and 0.2 gram dietary fiber. The same serving provides 15 percent of the RDA for vitamin A (150 RE), 6 percent of the RDA for folate (13 mcg), 1 percent of the RDA for niacin (0.2 mcg), 26 percent of the RDA for calcium (310 mg), and 12 percent of the RDA for magnesium (50 mg).

❖ **Selecting and storing.** Cocoa powder typically comes in an airtight metal container. Store in a cool, dry place, and choose dark cocoa for its high levels of heart-helping flavonoids.

 Kitchen Prescription

Dark and Decadent! Have a craving? Try our Chocolate Smoothie for a flavonoid fix.

Cranberries

Grown in bogs throughout Asia, Europe, and North America, these berries are best known for a Thanksgiving celebration and their ability to reduce the incidence of bladder infections. These tart treats contain flavonoids including anthocyanins that help to reduce total and LDL cholesterol and prevent LDL cholesterol from oxidizing.

❖ **Serving.** One cup of raw cranberries contains 46 calories, 0.4 gram protein, 12.1 grams carbohydrates, 0.2 gram fat, no cholesterol, and 4.4 grams dietary fiber. The same serving provides 21 percent of the RDA for vitamin C (12.8 mg). Cranberries also contain oxalic acid.

❖ **Selecting and storing.** Harvested between Labor Day and Halloween, the peak market period for cranberries is from October through December. They're usually packaged in twelve-ounce plastic bags. Any cranberries that are discolored or shriveled should be discarded. Cranberries can be refrigerated, tightly wrapped, for at least two months or frozen up to a year.

 Kitchen Prescription

Try our Apple and Cranberry Crisp for a delicious dessert full of phytonutrients!

Fish

Fish has been the subject of much research over the past twenty years since Danish researchers found a link between fish-eating Eskimos and low rates of heart disease. We now know that these sea creatures benefit the heart thanks to their omega-3 fatty acids and abundance of B vitamins.

❖ **Serving.** One serving of salmon (3 oz), baked or broiled, contains 149 calories, 20.5 grams protein, 0.4 gram carbohydrates, 6.8 grams fat, 35.7 milligrams cholesterol, and no dietary fiber. The same serving provides 122 percent of the RDA for niacin (24.5 mg), 115 percent of the RDA for vitamin B_{12} (2.3 mcg), and 20 percent of the RDA for phosphorus (238 mg).

❖ **Selecting and storing.** Choose fish with firm flesh that springs back with gentle pressure. The smell should be slightly briny, the gills should be moist and red, and the eyes should be clear and bright.

Healing Tip

Reel Health! Cold-water fish such as tuna, mackerel, herring, and sardines have higher amounts of omega-3s than do their warm-water kin. In fact, a 3½-ounce portion of sardines contains 5.1 grams of omega-3s, while the same portion size of chinook salmon contains 3 grams of omega-3s, Atlantic mackerel contains 2.2 grams of omega-3s, and pink salmon contains 1.9 grams of omega-3s. Troll our Fish and Seafood recipe section for perfect fish dishes.

Flaxseed

An ancient culinary staple used as early as 3000 B.C. and touted by Hippocrates, for its ability to relieve intestinal discomfort flaxseed has a mild nutty flavor and is often used simply sprinkled over hot dishes such as cooked cereal or stir-fry. This tiny seed provides heart-healthy omega-3 fatty acids and lignans that help to reduce total cholesterol while boosting HDL cholesterol levels.

✳ **Serving.** Two tablespoons of ground flaxseed contain 80 calories, 3.2 grams protein, no carbohydrates, 5.5 grams fat, no cholesterol, and 4.5 grams dietary fiber.

✳ **Selecting and storing.** Store flaxseed in the refrigerator or freezer, where it will keep for up to six months.

Healing Tip

The Daily Grind! Tap into the health benefits of flax with your coffee grinder. Its outer shell prevents many of the beneficial nutrients from being available, and grinding frees them up. Sprinkle over yogurt or cereal, or add to smoothies.

Garlic

A member of the allium, or onion, family, three major types of garlic are available in the United States: the white-skinned, strongly flavored American garlic; and the Mexican and Italian garlic—both of which have mauve-colored skins and a somewhat milder flavor. Elephant garlic (which is not a true garlic but a relative of the leek) is the most mildly flavored of the three. Garlic delivers cholesterol-reducing and heart-helping phytonutrients such as allicin, quercetin, and sulfides. In fact, as little as half a clove of garlic per day was found to decrease total serum cholesterol levels by 9 percent!

❖ **Serving.** One ounce of garlic contains no calories, protein, carbohydrates, fat, cholesterol, or fiber. It does contain 15 percent of vitamin B_6 and 15 percent of the RDA for vitamin C.

❖ **Selecting and storing.** Fresh garlic is available year-round. Purchase firm, plump bulbs with dry skins. Avoid heads with soft or shriveled cloves and those stored in the refrigerated section of the produce department. Store fresh garlic in an open container (away from other foods) in a cool, dark place. Properly stored, unbroken bulbs can be kept up to eight weeks, though they will begin to dry out toward the end of that time. Once broken from the bulb, individual cloves will keep for three to ten days.

 Kitchen Prescription

Get these cloves of protection in our Summer Vegetable Stew, but don't be afraid to add fresh pressed garlic to crusty whole-grain breads, salad dressings, or any of your favorite foods.

Grapefruit

A member of the citrus family of fruits grown in Florida, the grapefruit has been purported to be a weight-loss aid. Providing heart-helping flavonoids and cholesterol-lowering pectin and naringin, grapefruit falls on the low end of the GI scale. When you choose red grapefruit, you'll also get a dose of heart-protecting lycopene.

✤ **Serving.** One half grapefruit contains approximately 45 calories, 1 gram protein, 12 grams carbohydrates, 0.1 gram fat, no cholesterol, and 1.6 grams dietary fiber. The same serving provides 6 percent of the RDA for folate (11.8 mcg) and 66 percent of the RDA for vitamin C (39.3 mg).

✤ **Selecting and storing.** Fresh grapefruit is available year-round. Those from Arizona and California are in the market from about January through August; Florida and Texas grapefruits usually arrive around October and last through June. Choose grapefruits that have thin, fine-textured, brightly colored skin. They should be firm yet springy when held in the palm and pressed. Grapefruits keep best when wrapped in a plastic bag and placed in the vegetable drawer of the refrigerator for up to two weeks.

 Healing Tip

Culinary Caution! Grapefruit has numerous interactions with different medications (especially statins), so contact your doctor or pharmacist before consuming grapefruit if you take prescription medication.

Grapes

Grapes have been cultivated for as long as five thousand years and are classified as "European" (Thompson seedless, flame seedless, red globe) or "American" (Concord, Steuben, Delaware). The resveratrol found in the skins of red and white grapes plus quercetin help to reduce triglycerides and LDL cholesterol.

❖ **Serving.** One cup of raw European-type grapes, such as Thompson, contains 114 calories, 1.1 grams protein, 28.4 grams carbohydrates, 0.9 gram fat, no cholesterol, and 1.1 grams dietary fiber. The same serving provides 29 percent of the RDA for vitamin C (17.3 mg), 13 percent of the RDA for thiamin (0.2 mg), 10 percent of the RDA for vitamin B_6 (0.2 mg), 6 percent of the RDA for riboflavin (0.1 mg), and 296 milligrams potassium.

❖ **Selecting and storing.** Choose grapes that are plump, full-colored, and firmly attached to their stems. Green grapes should have a slight pale yellow hue, a sign of ripeness, while dark grapes should be deeply colored, with no sign of green. Store grapes unwashed in a plastic bag in the refrigerator for up to a week. Unless you buy organic, be sure to wash well as most grapes have been sprayed with insecticide.

 Healing Tip

Get the benefits of grapes fresh off the vine in red or purple grape juice or in red wine (in moderation).

Lemons

Citrus fruits cultivated in tropical and temperate climates around the world, lemons add zest and an abundance of vitamin C to foods and beverages. With cholesterol-lowering terpenes and antioxidant vitamin C, this tangy citrus falls low on the glycemic index.

❖ **Serving.** One tablespoon of lemon juice contains 4 calories, 0.1 gram protein, 1.4 grams carbohydrates, no fat, no cholesterol, and no dietary fiber. The same serving provides 11 percent of the RDA for vitamin C (75 mg).

❖ **Selecting and storing.** Lemons are available year-round, peaking during the summer months. Choose fruit with smooth, brightly colored skin with no tinge of green. Lemons should be firm, plump, and heavy for their size. Depending on their condition when purchased, they can be refrigerated in a plastic bag for two to three weeks.

 Kitchen Prescription

Have a "boca cocktail" to hydrate you through the day and deliver health-promoting phytonutrients. Just squeeze some fresh lemon into your spring water, and voilà!

Lentils

Members of the legume family, lentils come in red, green, and brown varieties. Phytoestrogens and fiber team up to make these high-protein morsels perfect for reducing cholesterol levels. They also deliver 86 percent of the RDA for folate—the B vitamin that helps to reduce levels of heart-harming homocysteine.

❖ **Serving.** One-half cup cooked lentils contains 101 calories, 9 grams protein, 18.4 grams carbohydrates, no fat, no cholesterol, and 9 grams dietary fiber. The same serving provides 86 percent of the RDA for folate (172.7 mcg), 15 percent of the RDA for iron (0.8 mg), and 7 percent of the RDA for thiamin (0.1 mg).

❖ **Selecting and storing.** Lentils should be stored in airtight containers at room temperature and will keep up to a year.

Kitchen Prescription

Love Your Legumes! Try our savory Lentil and Mushroom Soup for a light lunch or a first course to a heart-healthy meal.

Mangoes

Cultivated in India for several thousand years, mangoes come in hundreds of varieties. These tropical fruits are high in antioxidants, including vitamins C and E, plus carotenoids.

❖ **Serving.** One mango (about 7.3 oz) contains 128 calories, 1 gram protein, 33.4 grams carbohydrates, 0.57 gram fat, no cholesterol, and 3.7 grams dietary fiber. The same serving provides 90 percent of the RDA for vitamin C (54 mg), 77 percent of the RDA for vitamin A (766 RE), 24 percent of the RDA for vitamin E (2.4 mg), and 14 percent of the RDA for vitamin B_6 (0.28 mg).

❖ **Selecting and storing.** Mangoes are in season from May to September, though imported fruit is in the stores sporadically throughout the remainder of the year. Look for fruit with an unblemished yellow skin blushed with red.

Kitchen Prescription

Kick up the carotenoids with our Tropical Fruit Compote starring antioxidant-rich mango. It's a perfect choice for a delicious dessert that pleases the palate and protects the heart.

Nuts

Scientists speculate nuts may have been around tens of millions of years ago because they are native to both the Old World and the New. Cultivated for twelve thousand years, nuts are one of nature's richest foods. More than three hundred types of nuts exist, but those most commonly enjoyed include almonds, Brazil nuts, cashews, chestnuts, coconuts, hazelnuts, pecans, pistachios, walnuts, hickory nuts, pine nuts, and macadamia nuts. Full of minerals like copper and magnesium and packed with healthy fats and sterols, nuts also contain vitamin E to reduce the oxidation of LDL cholesterol. Although peanuts are actually a legume, research at Harvard School of Public Health and Penn State University has shown that peanuts reduce the risk of heart disease as well as type 2 diabetes. So don't be afraid to just go nuts!

❖ **Serving.** See individual packages of nuts for nutritional information.

❖ **Selecting and storing.** Store nuts in closed containers in the refrigerator or freezer to avoid rancidity. It is best to buy fresh raw nuts with shells, as they will store longer than shelled, cooked varieties.

 Healing Tip

Go Raw! Raw nuts contain more water to fill you up, and because they are not roasted, no oil or salt is added.

Oats

A highly rich-in-protein grain eaten in prepared cereals or as a hot cereal, oats are an American staple. The FDA awarded the first food-specific health claim to oats in January 1997 because of their ability to reduce total and LDL cholesterol. Compounds including tocotrienols, beta-glucan, and phytates may be to credit.

❖ **Serving.** One cup of cooked oatmeal (½ cup dry) contains 150 calories, 5.5 grams protein, 27 grams carbohydrates, 3 grams fat, no cholesterol, and 4 grams dietary fiber. The same serving size provides 13 percent of the RDA for thiamin (0.2 mg), 31 percent of the RDA for magnesium (107 mg), and 9 percent of the RDA for iron (1.9 mg).

❖ **Selecting and storing.** Store oats in a cool, dry place and choose steel-cut oats, as they are the most nutritious and least processed.

 Kitchen Prescription

Get these heart-healthy grains in our Cinnamon Raisin Scones.

Olive Oil

Most olive oil comes from California, and it is also imported from France, Greece, Italy, and Spain. It is made by pressing tree-ripened olives to extract a flavorful, heart-healthy monounsaturated oil that is prized throughout the world both for cooking and for putting on salads. The flavor, color, and fragrance of olive oils can vary depending on distinctions such as growing region and the crop's condition. Olive oil is also rich in phenolic compounds and oleic acid, which benefit the heart. All olive oils are graded in accordance with their degree of acidity. The best are cold-pressed, a chemical-free process that involves only pressure, which produces a natural level of low acidity. Extra-virgin olive oil, the cold-pressed result of the first pressing of the olives, is only 1 percent acid. It is considered the finest and fruitiest of the olive oils and is therefore also the most expensive. It can range from a champagne color to greenish-golden to bright green.

✤ **Serving.** One tablespoon of extra-virgin olive oil contains 120 calories, no protein, no carbohydrates, 14 grams fat, no cholesterol, and no dietary fiber.

✤ **Selecting and storing.** Olive oil should be stored in a cool, dark place for up to six months. It can be refrigerated, in which case it will last up to a year.

 Healing Tip

In general, the deeper the color, the more intense the olive flavor and the more phytonutrients present.

Onions

Members of the allium family, onions have two main classifications: green onions and dry onions, which are simply mature onions with a juicy flesh covered with dry, papery skin. With their cholesterol-reducing sulfur compounds and quercetin, onions add flavor and health to any dish.

✤ **Serving.** One medium raw onion contains 60 calories, 2 grams protein, 14 grams carbohydrates, no fat, no cholesterol, and 3 grams dietary fiber. The same serving also provides 18 percent of the RDA for vitamin C (12 mg).

✤ **Selecting and storing.** When buying onions, choose those that are heavy for their size with dry, papery skins and no signs of spotting or moistness. Avoid onions with soft spots. Store in a cool, dry place with good air circulation for up to two months (depending on their condition when purchased). Once cut, an onion should be tightly wrapped, refrigerated, and used within four days.

Kitchen Prescription

You'll find these tearful treats in many of our recipes. Toss them into salads, dice and sauté into sauces, or chop and add to soups. Experiment with different varieties of onions such as cippolini, Texas onions, Vidalia onions, and shallots.

Oranges

The most popular citrus fruit, oranges are believed to have originated in Southeast Asia and been brought to the New World by Christopher Columbus. A low-GI food, oranges pack a powerful punch of antioxidant vitamin C, some vitamin A, plus a bevy of cholesterol-reducing flavonoids including hesperidin, naringin, and nobiletin. Refer back to Chapter 4 to see how citrus helps conquer cholesterol.

❖ **Serving.** One orange (approximately 4.6 oz) contains 62 calories, 1.3 grams protein, 15.4 grams carbohydrates, 0.2 gram fat, no cholesterol, and 3 grams dietary fiber. The same serving provides 20 percent of the RDA for folate (39.7 mcg), 92 percent of the RDA for vitamin C (69.7 mg), 13 percent of the RDA for thiamin (0.2 mg), 4 percent of the RDA for calcium (52 mg), and 237 milligrams potassium.

❖ **Selecting and storing.** Fresh oranges are available year-round at different times, depending on the variety. Choose fruit that is firm and heavy for its size, with no mold or spongy spots. Oranges can be stored at cool room temperature for a day or so but should then be refrigerated and kept there for up to two weeks.

Kitchen Prescription

Kick up the carotenoids with our Carotene Cooler starring this sunny citrus fruit. It's a perfect choice for breakfast served with high-fiber, whole-grain cereal.

Peaches

Widely planted across the eastern seaboard by the early settlers, many botanists thought peaches were indigenous to the United States. The peach is the third most popular of all fruits grown in the United States and comes in numerous varieties. With their flavonoids and carotenoids, peaches are sweet on the heart and on the palate.

❖ **Serving.** One peach (approximately 4 oz) contains 37 calories, 0.7 gram protein, 9.7 grams carbohydrates, 0.1 gram fat, no cholesterol, and 1.5 grams dietary fiber. The same serving also provides 47 percent of the RDA for vitamin A (465 RE), 19 percent of the RDA for vitamin C (1.7 mg), and 8 percent of the RDA for niacin (1.5 mg).

❖ **Selecting and storing.** Peaches are available from May to October in most regions of the United States. Look for fragrant fruit that gives slightly to palm pressure. Avoid those with signs of greening.

 Kitchen Prescription

Enjoy these fuzzy fruits ripe off the tree or in our Peach and Berry Tart.

Peppers

Part of the nightshade family of vegetables, many varieties of peppers exist including banana, red bell, yellow bell, green bell, chili, cayenne, jalapeño, habanero, and Scotch bonnet. Along with heart-helping vitamin C and magnesium, if you choose red peppers you'll also get a dose of lycopene—a powerful compound that helps reduce the oxidation of LDL cholesterol that contributes to heart disease.

❖ **Serving.** One-half cup red bell pepper contains 14 calories, 0.5 gram protein, 3.2 grams carbohydrates, 0.1 gram fat, no cholesterol, and 1.8 grams dietary fiber. The same serving also provides 11 percent of the RDA for folate (22.2 mcg), 44 percent of the RDA for vitamin C (26.1 mg), 35 percent of the RDA for vitamin B_6 (0.7 mg), 17 percent of the RDA for niacin (3.3 mg), 18 percent of the RDA for thiamin (0.2 mg), 14 percent of the RDA for magnesium (54.5 mg), 19 percent of the RDA for iron (2.8 mg), and 844 milligrams potassium.

❖ **Selecting and storing.** Choose peppers that are firm; have a brightly colored, shiny skin; and are heavy for their size. Avoid those that are limp, shriveled, or have soft or bruised spots. Store peppers in a plastic bag in the refrigerator for up to a week.

 Kitchen Prescription

Saucy Protection! Try our Broiled Mahimahi with Red Bell Pepper Sauce for a unique twist on a traditional fish dish.

Pomegranates

Pomegranates are unusual fruits with bright red juice and many seeds. The name comes from two French words, *pome* and *granate*, and literally means "apple with many seeds." These unique fruits provide a good dose of fiber plus anthocyanins that halt the oxidation of LDL cholesterol, reduce the stickiness of platelets, and help reduce LDL.

❖ **Serving.** One pomegranate (approximately 5.5 oz) contains 104 calories, 1.5 grams protein, 26.5 grams carbohydrates, 0.5 gram fat, no cholesterol, and 1 gram dietary fiber. The same serving also provides 16 percent of the RDA for vitamin C (9.4 mg) and 399 milligrams potassium.

❖ **Selecting and storing.** In the United States pomegranates are available in October and November. Choose those that are heavy for their size and have a bright, fresh color and blemish-free skin. Refrigerate for up to two months, or store in a cool, dark place for up to a month.

 Kitchen Prescription

Sprinkle pomegranate buds over your favorite cereal or try pomegranate juice mixed with sparking mineral water for a refreshing beverage.

Pumpkins

A flowering vegetable and member of the gourd family, pumpkins are powerhouses of carotenoids to be enjoyed year-round.

❖ **Serving.** One-half cup of canned pumpkin contains 41 calories, 1.3 grams protein, 9.9 grams carbohydrates, 0.3 gram fat, no cholesterol, and 3.6 grams dietary fiber. The same serving also provides 269 percent of the RDA for vitamin A (2,691 RE), 8 percent of the RDA for folate (15 mcg), 9 percent of the RDA for vitamin C (5.1 mg), 11 percent of the RDA for iron (1.7 mg), 7 percent of the RDA for magnesium (28 mg), and 251 milligrams potassium.

❖ **Selecting and storing.** Fresh pumpkins are available in the fall and winter, and some specimens have weighed in at well over a hundred pounds. In general, however, the flesh from smaller sizes will be more tender and succulent. Choose pumpkins that are free from blemishes and heavy for their size. Store whole pumpkins at room temperature up to a month, or refrigerate up to three months.

 Kitchen Prescription

Don't put these gorgeous gourds off until Thanksgiving! Buy canned pumpkin and mix it into smoothies, muffins, and pancakes. For perfect pumpkin recipes, visit healinggourmet.com.

Raspberries

Typically red, raspberries also come in other colors such as purple, yellow, amber, and black. These antioxidant-rich berries provide cholesterol-cutting flavonoids—including anthocyanins—plus antioxidant vitamin C.

❖ **Serving.** One cup of raspberries contains 61 calories, 1.2 grams protein, 14.3 grams carbohydrates, 0.7 gram fat, no cholesterol, and 8 grams dietary fiber. The same serving also provides 16 percent of the RDA for folate (32 mcg), 51 percent of the RDA for vitamin C (30.8 mg), 6 percent of the RDA for magnesium (22 mg), and 5 percent of the RDA for iron (0.7 mg).

✤ **Selecting and storing.** Raspberries are available from May through November. Choose brightly colored, plump berries without the hull. If the hulls are still attached, the berries were picked too early and will undoubtedly be tart. Avoid soft, shriveled, or moldy berries. Store in a dry container in the refrigerator for two to three days. If necessary, rinse lightly just before serving.

 Kitchen Prescription

Our Berry Blast is a quick and delicious way to get your daily dose of raspberries. For a morning smoothie or a post-workout refresher, this delightful drink is full of flavorful flavonoids!

Soybeans

Members of the legume family and a complete protein, soybeans are a main staple of the Asian diet. Scientists are discovering that compounds including phytoestrogens, isoflavones, and saponins are to credit for the soybeans cholesterol-reducing and heart-helping benefits.

✤ **Serving.** One-quarter block of tofu (approximately 4 oz) contains 90 calories, 9.4 grams protein, 2.2 grams carbohydrates, 5.4 grams fat, no cholesterol, and 1.4 grams dietary fiber. The same serving provides 30 percent of the RDA for magnesium (120 mg), 41 percent of the RDA for iron (6.2 mg), and 10 percent of the RDA for calcium (122 mg).

✤ **Selecting and storing.** Experiment with the many different varieties of soy foods. *Edamame* are soybeans in their shell, and they can be found in the freezer section of your grocery and stored in the pod or found in the refrigerator case, cooked and out of their shells. *Tempeh* is soybean curd that has a meaty texture and can also be found in the refrigerator case. *Textured veg-*

etable protein (*TVP*) is processed soy that has the consistency of ground meat. It can be used in chilies, sauces, soups, or anywhere you would use ground meat; it is available in either the dry section of your grocery or in the freezer section. *Tofu* is very perishable and should be refrigerated for no more than a week. If it's packaged in water, drain it and cover with fresh water and change the water daily. Tofu can be frozen up to three months.

 Kitchen Prescription

All soy foods take on the flavors you cook them with, so make liberal use of those phytonutrient herbs and spices when cooking with soy products. Our Fajita Burgers deliver a mouthwatering dose of soy protein. Serve with sweet potato "fries" for a healthy twist on an all-American classic.

Spinach

A leafy green native of Asia, spinach was brought to Europe by the Moors when they conquered Spain in the eighth century. Spinach provides a healthy dose of folate—to help reduce heart-harming homocysteine—plus carotenoids, lutein, and zeaxanthin. Refer back to Chapter 4 for more on these fabulous phytonutrients.

✳ **Serving.** One-half cup of cooked spinach contains 21 calories, 2.7 grams protein, 3.4 grams carbohydrates, 0.2 gram fat, no cholesterol, and 2.1 grams dietary fiber. The same serving provides 74 percent of the RDA for vitamin A (737 RE), 66 percent of the RDA for folate (131.2 mcg), 20 percent of the RDA for magnesium (78.3 mg), 21 percent of the RDA for iron (3.2 mg), and 10 percent of the RDA for calcium (122.4 mg).

✳ **Selecting and storing.** Fresh spinach is available year-round. Choose leaves that are crisp and dark green with a nice fresh fragrance. Avoid those that are limp or damaged or have yellow spots. Refrigerate in a plastic bag for up to three days. Spinach, which is usually very gritty, must be thoroughly rinsed.

Kitchen Prescription

Our Sole Florentine combines vitamin B–rich fish with full-of-folate spinach for a heart-healthy flavor you'll get hooked on!

Strawberries

Strawberries are the most popular American berry, and more than seventy varieties of this nutrient-rich food exist. With their red color, these boisterous berries boast lycopene in their disease-fighting arsenal.

❖ **Serving.** One cup of raw strawberries contains 45 calories, 1 gram protein, 10.5 grams carbohydrates, 0.6 gram fat, no cholesterol, and 2.9 grams dietary fiber. The same serving provides 13 percent of the RDA for folate (26.4 mg), 141 percent of the RDA for vitamin C (84.5 mg), 4 percent of the RDA for iron (0.6 mg), and 247 milligrams potassium.

❖ **Selecting and storing.** Fresh strawberries are available year-round in many regions of the country, with the peak season from April to June. Choose brightly colored, plump berries that still have their leaves attached. Avoid soft, shriveled, or moldy berries. Do not wash until ready to use, and store in a dry container in the refrigerator for two to three days.

Kitchen Prescription

Use strawberries in our Peach and Berry Tart for a healthy dessert that's delicious for your heart!

Tea

Used by the ancient Chinese, the Greeks, medieval herbalists, and scholars of the Enlightenment for their medicinal purposes, black tea, green tea, and oolong tea come from the *Camellia sinensis* plant. Phytonutrients in tea—such as catechins and tannins—help to reduce cholesterol, boost antioxidant levels in the blood, and reduce the risk of a dangerous clot.

✣ **Serving.** Six ounces of black tea contain 2 calories, no protein, 0.5 gram carbohydrates, no fat, no cholesterol, and no dietary fiber. The same serving provides 5 percent of the RDA for folate (1 mcg).

✣ **Selecting and storing.** Store tea bags or loose tea in an airtight container in a cool dry place.

 Kitchen Prescription

Try our Zesty Green Tea Cooler or Spicy Cinnamon Chai. Don't forget to let your tea steep at least two minutes to get the full benefit of those phytonutrients!

Tomatoes

Thought to have originated from South America, tomatoes were brought by Spanish explorers to Europe in the 1500s. Most notable for their lycopene, tomatoes help to protect the heart by reducing oxidation of LDL cholesterol.

✣ **Serving.** One red, ripe tomato (approximately 4.3 oz) contains 24 calories, 1.1 grams protein, 5.3 grams carbohydrates, 0.3 gram fat, no cholesterol, and 1.3 grams dietary fiber. The same serving provides 14 percent of the RDA for vitamin A (139 RE), 6 percent of the RDA for folate (11.6 mcg), 36 percent of the RDA for vitamin C (21.6 mg), and 5 percent of the RDA for iron (0.8 mg).

❖ **Selecting and storing.** Choose firm, well-shaped tomatoes that are fragrant and richly colored (for their variety). They should be free from blemishes, be heavy for their size, and give slightly to pressure. Ripe tomatoes should be stored at room temperature and used within a few days, as cold temperatures make the flesh pithy.

 Kitchen Prescription

Cooking tomatoes helps to unlock lycopene, a fat-soluble antioxidant nutrient. Adding a bit of oil also helps aid in the absorption. Get out the saucepan!

Wheat

One of the oldest grains cultivated, wheat is available in numerous forms including berries, cracked wheat, bulgur grits, shredded wheat, unprocessed bran (or miller's bran), wheat germ, rolled wheat flakes, puffed wheat, cream of wheat, and wheat flour.

❖ **Serving.** One slice of whole-wheat bread contains 90 calories, 4 grams protein, 15 grams carbohydrates, 1 gram fat, no cholesterol, and 3 grams dietary fiber. The same serving provides 2 percent of the RDA for folate (4.1 mcg), 6 percent of the RDA for niacin (1.2 mg), 6 percent of the RDA for thiamin (0.09 mg), and 2 percent of the RDA for riboflavin (0.04 mg).

❖ **Selecting and storing.** Whole-wheat flour contains part of the grain's germ and turns rancid quickly because of the oil in the germ. Refrigerate or freeze these flours tightly wrapped, and use as soon as possible.

Healing Tip

Don't forget to look for the words *whole grain* when buying wheat. Whole-grain products have not been "refined" or stripped of their nutritious germ and bran layers, which help to keep cholesterol levels in check.

So far we've examined the various nutritional elements in different foods and diets. Next, you'll learn which herbs and spices you should be stocking in your kitchen.

Healing Herbs
and Spices

THE FRAGRANT SMELL of basil in our recipe for Pesto Salmon
or the cinnamon-scented steam wafting from our Spicy Cinnamon Chai does more than please the palate and perfume the air.
Nature's flavor enhancers are endowed with an abundance of—
what else?—phytonutrients! Researchers at the Cytokine Research
Laboratory, Department of Experimental Therapeutics at the
University of Texas uniquely describe this as the "reasoning for
seasoning." In this chapter we discuss some of the herbs and spices
that can lower cholesterol and the phytonutrients responsible for
their delicious protection (as seen in Table 6.1). We also give you
tips on how to use them with the recipes from Chapter 9 to create heart-healthy meals that heal!

Savoring Flavor

The liberal use of fragrant spices and herbs is not a new concept.
For centuries these flavor enhancers have been used to boost cuisine, treat illnesses, and prevent spoilage. In ancient times, people prized spices more highly than gold or jewels. In today's world
of high-sodium and high-fat processed foods, consumers are turning back to herbs and spices to add flavor and zest to their meals.

TABLE 6.1 Cholesterol-Cutting Herbs and Spices

Herb/Spice Family	Member	Phytochemicals
Labitae (mint family)	Basil, mint, oregano, rosemary, sage, thyme	Terpenoids, menthol, and chlorophyll
Umbelliferae (umbel family)	Anise, caraway, carrots, celeriac, celery, chervil, cilantro, coriander, cumin, dill, fennel, parsley, parsnips	Carotenoids, beta-carotene, alpha-carotene, beta-cryptoxanthin, zeaxanthin, lutein, chlorophyll
Zingiberaceae (ginger family)	Ginger, turmeric	Curcumin, gingerols, zingibain

Using nature's flavor enhancers delivers an abundance of heart-helping phytonutrients while eliminating added calories and salt. You can refer back to Chapter 4 to discover how each of these phytonutrients works as part of a team to reduce cholesterol and protect the heart.

A Spice Rack That Lowers Cholesterol

Unlike herbs, which come from the leaves of plants, spices are made from the buds, barks, fruits, seeds, or roots. Although research of the healing powers of spices is relatively new, what scientists have discovered thus far has been impressive. Rich in phytonutrients and antioxidants, spice varieties have been found to reduce cholesterol, keep the arteries clear, stabilize blood sugar, and fight many chronic illnesses including cancer. Not unlike the other plant foods we eat, the colors indicate how these flavor enhancers work in our bodies to protect our cardiac muscle and cut cholesterol. Most spices—including cinnamon, bay leaves, allspice, and cloves—help to protect our heart through their antioxidant and anti-inflammatory action and beneficial effects on blood sugar. Be sure to store your spices in a cool, dark place to preserve their potency and enhance shelf life. Let's take a look at the individual spices to include in your rack!

 Healing Tip

Boost the flavor of spices by toasting them briefly in a dry skillet until slightly brown and aromatic.

Allspice. Allspice is the dried, unripe berry of *Pimenta dioica*—an evergreen tree in the myrtle family. After drying, the berries are small, dark brown balls just a little larger than peppercorns. Allspice comes from Jamaica, Mexico, and Honduras. Pungent and fragrant, it is not a blend of "all spices," but its taste and aroma remind many people of a mix of cloves, cinnamon, and nutmeg.

 Healing Tip

Allspice is used in Jamaican jerk seasoning and in Jamaican soups, stews, and curries. It also is used in pickling spice, spiced tea mixes, cakes, cookies, and pies.

Anise. A gray-brown oval seed from *Pimpinella anisum*, a plant in the Umbelliferae or carrot family, anise is related to caraway, dill, cumin, and fennel. Spain and Mexico are the sources for anise, although it is native to the Middle East.

Healing Tip

You can use anise in cakes, cookies, and sweet breads like Europeans do, or in soups and stews as is done in the Middle East and India.

Bay Leaves. Bay leaves come from the sweet bay or laurel tree, known botanically as *Laurus nobilis*. The elliptical leaves of both trees are green, glossy, and grow up to three inches long. Grown in the Mediterranean region and a staple in American kitchens, bay leaves are used in soups, stews, and meat and vegetable dishes. The leaves also flavor classic French dishes such as bouillabaisse.

Kitchen Prescription

Taste bay leaves in our Lentil and Mushroom Soup.

Cinnamon. Cinnamon is the dried bark of various laurel trees in the cinnamomun family. The cinnamon used in North America is from the cassia tree, which is grown in Vietnam, China, Indonesia, and Central America. Cinnamon has a sweet, woody fragrance in both ground and stick forms that enhances the taste of vegetables and fruits.

Kitchen Prescription

Our Cinnamon Raisin Scones are a delicious way to get your dose of this spice.

Cloves. Cloves are the rich, brown, dried, unopened flower buds of *Syzygium aromaticum*, an evergreen tree in the myrtle family. The name comes from the French *clou*, meaning nail. Cloves come from Madagascar, Brazil, Panang, and Ceylon and are strong, pungent, and sweet.

Kitchen Prescription

Get cloves in our recipe for Indian Spice Mix (from Chapter 4), and add it to chicken, fish, and bean dishes.

Cumin. Cumin is the pale green seed of *Cuminum cyminum*, a small herb in the Umbelliferae or carrot family. The seed is uniformly elliptical and deeply furrowed, frequently used in Mexican dishes, and has a distinctive, slightly bitter yet warm flavor.

Kitchen Prescription

Find this spice in our Black Bean Burritos.

Fennel. Fennel seed is the oval, green or yellowish-brown dried fruit of *Foeniculum vulgare*, a member of the Umbelliferae or carrot family. Fennel goes well with fish and is used in some curry powder mixes. Fennel has an anise-like flavor but is more aromatic, sweeter, and less pungent.

Kitchen Prescription

Try this unforgettable flavor in our Mediterranean Baked Snapper.

Ginger. A member of the Zingiberacae family—which includes turmeric—ginger comes mainly from Jamaica, India, Africa, and China. With a peppery and slightly sweet flavor and a spicy and pungent aroma, this extremely versatile root has long been a mainstay in Asian and Indian cooking and found its way early on into European foods as well. Compounds in ginger called *gingerols* have clot-busting action and have also been found to prevent the oxidation of LDL cholesterol that increases the risk for heart disease. Young ginger, often called spring ginger, has a pale, thin skin that requires no peeling. Mature ginger has a tough skin that must be peeled away to reveal the delicate flesh just under the surface.

 Kitchen Prescription

Look for ginger with smooth skin and a fresh, spicy fragrance. Fresh, unpeeled gingerroot, tightly wrapped, can be refrigerated for up to three weeks and frozen for up to six months. Try it in our Carrot Ginger Bisque.

Saffron. The stigma of *Crocus sativus*, a flowering plant in the crocus family and native to the Mediterranean, saffron is the world's most expensive spice; more than 225,000 stigmas must be hand-picked to produce one pound. In its pure form, saffron is a mass of compressed, threadlike, dark orange strands. Primarily cultivated in Spain, saffron has a spicy, pungent, and bitter flavor with a sharp and penetrating odor.

 Healing Tip

You can use saffron in French bouillabaisse, Spanish paella, and many Middle Eastern dishes.

Turmeric. Turmeric comes from the root of *Curcuma longa*, a leafy plant in the Zingiberaceae or ginger family. The root, or rhizome, has a tough brown skin and bright orange flesh. Ground turmeric comes from fingers, which extend from the root. It is boiled or steamed and then dried and ground. India is the world's primary producer of turmeric, but it is also grown in China and Indonesia. Studies show that turmeric may help to reduce blood cholesterol levels. It is mildly aromatic, has scents of orange or ginger, and has a pungent, bitter flavor.

 Healing Tip

Turmeric is a necessary ingredient of curry powder and is used extensively in Indian dishes—including lentil and meat dishes—and in Southeast Asian cooking.

Herbs for Health

Prior to the discovery of modern pharmaceuticals, both Europeans and Americans relied on herbs to treat illness and promote health. Researchers now know that the phytonutrients in herbs provide a range of health benefits, including working as part of your cholesterol-cutting team of plant foods. Although numerous healing herbs exist, we will focus on some of the most common culinary herbs that bring aroma to your kitchen and an added dose of health to your meals.

Basil. A bright green, leafy plant (*Ocimum basilicum*) in the Labitae or mint family, basil is grown primarily in the United States, France, and the Mediterranean region. Basil is widely used in Italian cuisine (often paired with tomatoes) and is also used in Thai cooking. Basil has a sweet, herbal bouquet, and its name means "be fragrant."

Kitchen Prescription

Try our Marinated Provençale Salad to get this delicious herb.

Cilantro. The leaf of the young coriander plant (*Coriandrum sativum*), cilantro is an herb in the Umbelliferae or carrot family—similar to anise. Grown in California and traditionally used in Middle Eastern, Mexican, and Asian cooking, cilantro's taste is a fragrant mix of parsley and citrus.

Kitchen Prescription

Try this unique-flavored herb in our Wild Rice Salad.

Dill. This tall, feathery annual (*Anethum graveolens*) is in the Umbelliferae or carrot family. Both dill seed and weed (dried leaves) come from the same plant and are widely used in pickling as well as in German, Russian, and Scandinavian dishes. The dill seed flavor is clean, pungent, and reminiscent of caraway, though dill weed has a similar but mellower and fresher flavor.

Kitchen Prescription

Our Greek Orzo and Shrimp Salad makes delicious use of dill.

Marjoram. Marjoram is the gray-green leaf of *Majorana hortensis*, a low-growing member of the Labitae or mint family. Often mistaken for oregano, marjoram has a delicate, sweet, pleasant flavor with a slightly bitter undertone.

Kitchen Prescription

Try marjoram in our Marinated Provençale Salad.

Mint. Mint is the dried leaf of a perennial herb in the Labitae family. There are two important species: *Mentha spicata L.* (spearmint) and *Mentha piperita L.* (peppermint).

 Kitchen Prescription

Try our Tropical Fruit Compote with mint.

Oregano. Oregano is the dried leaf of *Origanum vulgare L.*, a perennial herb in the Labitae or mint family. Mexican oregano is the dried leaf of one of several plants of the *Lippia* genus. Grown in California and New Mexico, as well as in the Mediterranean region, oregano is the spice that gives pizza its characteristic flavor. It is also usually used in chili powder. Oregano has a pungent odor and flavor with the Mexican variety being a bit stronger than Mediterranean oregano.

 Kitchen Prescription

Get fragrant oregano in our Zesty Lemon Chicken.

Parsley. Parsley is a member of the Umbelliferae or carrot family and is commonly used as a flavoring and garnish. Although more than thirty varieties of this herb exist, the most popular are curly leaf parsley and the more strongly flavored Italian or flat-leaf parsley.

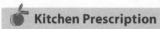 **Kitchen Prescription**

Our Middle Eastern Bulgur Salad makes liberal use of parsley.

Rosemary. Rosemary is an herb in the Labitae or mint family. A small evergreen shrub native to the Mediterranean, the leaves of *Rosmarinus officinalis* resemble curved pine needles. Today it is widely produced in France, Spain, and Portugal and has a distinct tealike aroma and a piney flavor. Rosemary contains rosmarinic acid, among other phytonutrients, which help to reduce inflammatory factors involved with the development of heart disease and other chronic illnesses.

 Kitchen Prescription

Try rosemary in our Lentil and Mushroom Soup.

Sage. An herb from an evergreen shrub *Salvia officinalis*, in the Labitae or mint family, sage's long, grayish-green leaves take on a velvety, cottonlike texture when rubbed (meaning they are ground lightly and passed through a coarse sieve). Grown primarily in the United States as well as in Dalmatia and Albania, sage has a fragrant aroma and an astringent but warm flavor. The name "sage" comes from the Latin word *salia*, meaning "to save."

Thyme. Thyme is the leaf of a low-growing shrub in the Labitae or mint family called *Thymus vulgaris*. Its tiny grayish-green leaves are rarely greater than one-fourth inch long. For use as a condiment, thyme leaves are dried and then chopped or ground. Grown in southern Europe, including France, Spain, and Portugal, thyme is also indigenous to the Mediterranean. Thyme has a subtle, dry aroma and a slightly minty flavor.

Kitchen Prescription

Take the time to try thyme in our Summer Vegetable Stew.

Perfect Pairings

Now that we have explored some of the healing properties of herbs and spices, let's take a look at the flavor combinations that please the palate. Don't be afraid to experiment and create your own blends to design savory and healthy meals.

* **Poultry.** Rosemary and thyme; tarragon, marjoram, and garlic; cumin, bay leaf, and saffron (or turmeric); ginger, cinnamon, and allspice; curry powder and thyme
* **Fish and seafood.** Cumin and oregano; tarragon, thyme, parsley, and garlic; thyme, fennel, saffron, and red pepper; ginger, sesame, and white pepper; cilantro, parsley, cumin, and garlic
* **Beans.** Marjoram and rosemary; caraway and dry mustard
* **Broccoli.** Ginger and garlic; sesame and nutmeg
* **Cabbage.** Celery seeds and dill; curry powder and nutmeg
* **Carrots.** Cinnamon and nutmeg; ginger
* **Corn.** Chili powder and cumin; dill
* **Peas.** Anise; rosemary and marjoram
* **Spinach.** Curry powder and ginger; nutmeg and garlic
* **Summer squash.** Mint and parsley; tarragon and garlic
* **Winter squash.** Cinnamon and nutmeg; allspice and red pepper
* **Tomatoes.** Basil and rosemary; cinnamon and ginger
* **Potatoes.** Dill and parsley; caraway; nutmeg and chives
* **Rice.** Chili powder and cumin; curry powder, ginger, and coriander; cinnamon, cardamom, and cloves

❖ **Pasta.** Basil, rosemary, and parsley; cumin, turmeric, and red pepper; oregano and thyme

Now that you've filled your spice rack with healing herbs and spices, in the next chapter, we offer tips for other items to put into your shopping cart to lower cholesterol and prevent heart disease.

7

Shopping for Health

THE FIRST STEP to a healthy heart is making wise choices in the grocery and when dining out. Unfortunately, with so many products on the market, selecting healthful items to stock your pantry and choose in a restaurant can be a daunting task. In this chapter, we give you practical tips on becoming a grocery and dining guru to cut your cholesterol. Healing Gourmet will help you decipher food labels and the art of shopping for health.

Strategies for Smart Shopping

Understanding the science behind how foods can protect us is useful only if we can translate that information into our grocery carts and ultimately onto our tables. Because most of us spend a substantial amount of time at the grocery (84 percent of consumers prepare home-cooked meals at least three times a week), it is critical to navigate the supermarket smorgasbord to find the healthiest products.

Before you go to the store, make a list and check it twice. Smart shopping begins before you leave the house. Being unprepared leads to multiple trips and unwanted, often unhealthy, items finding their way into your shopping cart. Instead of buying on impulse, stray from your list only if the item is a healthy one. If junior shoppers vying for the candy aisle accompany you, have them explore the produce section and let them choose a unique fruit or vegetable to try (e.g., a persimmon, pomegranate, or kiwi fruit) to foster good health habits. Also, before you venture to the grocery store, you should eat. Shopping hungry is a surefire way to end up straying from your list and succumbing to unhealthy choices. Having a small snack will help you to avoid temptations that will wind up in your cupboard and on your waist.

When filling your cart, become a perimeter shopper. The exterior of the store contains many of the whole foods we have described for optimum health. Spend most of your time shopping for fresh produce, seafood, lean meats, and dairy. When choosing dairy, opt for lower-calorie products such as shredded mozzarella, low-fat soft cheeses, and yogurt as opposed to aged, hard cheeses such as cheddar—which rack up 100 calories for each one-ounce cube.

There is so much variation in the health value of different brands of foods, so it's important to pause, read labels, and compare choices. Read ingredient lists and look at calories and sugar, the types of grains used (whole grains vs. refined), and the types of oils used (partially hydrogenated vegetable oil vs. olive oil or canola oil). We will demystify the food label later in this chapter.

What to Look for When Selecting Ingredients

It's easy to incorporate all the cholesterol-lowering foods, herbs, and spices plus the "healthy fats" and "healthy carbs" we talked about in earlier chapters. Remember those colors we described in Chapter 5? You want to look for those same colors to put them in your cart and build your meals around them. Also, as we mentioned in Chapter 6, the condiment aisle is a good place to find products that are full of flavor and a great way to add zesty phytonutrient protection to your meals. Go back to that chapter, and make sure you have the right herbs and spices in your kitchen. In addition, purchase high-quality cooking oils such as extra-virgin olive oil, sesame oil, expeller-pressed canola oil, and other liquid vegetable oils for sautéing and adding to dressings and marinades. Buy mustard, vinegars, horseradish, and the dried herbs and spices that help prevent and manage diabetes and add virtually no calories and lots of flavor to all varieties of foods.

Shopping for Meat, Poultry, Fish, and Other Sources of Protein

Choose only the leanest meats and poultry to help you lower your cholesterol. Because even the leanest meat, chicken, and fish have saturated fat and cholesterol, limit the total amount you eat. It's also a good idea to avoid the deli when shopping. Although many deli foods are marketed as "fresh," most are processed red meats or poultry, which can have a dangerous effect on the heart and cholesterol levels. Some chicken and turkey hot dogs are lower in saturated fat than pork and beef hot dogs. There are also "lean" beef hot dogs and vegetarian (made with tofu) franks that are low in saturated fat.

When shopping for poultry remember that the white meat itself always contains less saturated fat than the dark meat. Try fresh ground turkey or chicken that is made from white meat such as the breast. In addition, chicken and turkey are low in saturated fat—especially when the skin is removed—so choose chicken and turkey without skin or remove the skin before eating. You should also limit goose and duck as they are high in saturated fat—even with the skin removed.

Most fish (such as cod) are lower in saturated fat than meat or poultry. Try to include fatty fish each week to provide heart-healthy omega-3s. Also, keep in mind that while shellfish have little saturated fat and total fat, they vary in cholesterol content.

In addition, meat substitutes, such as dry peas, dry beans, and tofu (bean curd), are great meat substitutes that are low in saturated fat and provide an abundance of phytonutrients. Dry peas and beans also have a lot of fiber, which can help to lower blood cholesterol. Try adding a half cup of beans to pasta, soups, casseroles, and vegetable dishes. Tofu takes on the flavor of whatever you marinate it with; try marinating it in a nonfat dressing or a tangy sauce and grilling or baking for a heart-healthy dish.

Finally, go nuts for your health! Instead of chips, pretzels, and other nutrient-void snack foods, opt for raw or roasted nuts and seeds, which are full of minerals, good-quality fats, and other health-promoting nutrients. Just be sure to watch your portion size: a quarter cup of almonds, for example, contains 170 calories.

What to Get in the Dairy Aisle

Like high-fat meats, regular dairy foods that have fat—such as whole and 2 percent milk, cheese, and ice cream—are also high in saturated fat.

Egg yolks are high in dietary cholesterol, as each contains about 213 milligrams. Whole eggs can be part of a healthy diet but should be limited to three per week. Egg whites, on the other hand, have no cholesterol, and you can substitute them for whole eggs in recipes (two egg whites are equal to one whole egg). You can also use cholesterol-free egg substitute in place of whole eggs. In many baked goods, you can't tell the difference.

When shopping for milk, buy fat-free and 1 percent milk rather than whole or 2 percent milk. Fat-free and 1 percent milk have just as much or more calcium and other nutrients as whole milk—with much less saturated fat.

When looking for hard cheeses, go for the versions that are "fat free," "reduced fat," "low fat," or "part skim." Choose varieties that have 2 grams of fat or less per ounce. When looking for soft cheeses, choose low-fat (1 percent) or nonfat cottage cheese, farmer cheese, or part-skim or light ricotta. Some of these cheeses have 2 grams of fat or less per ounce. If you are watching your sodium intake, choose lower-sodium cheeses. (Read the label to compare the sodium content.)

Buy low-fat or nonfat yogurt; like many other dairy foods, it is an excellent source of protein and calcium. Eat low-fat or non-fat yogurt alone or as a topping or in recipes. Try topping with fruit. In addition, try low-fat or nonfat sour cream or cream cheese blends. Many taste as rich as the real thing but have less fat and calories.

Fruits and Vegetables

When you look in your shopping cart, the vast majority of your food selection should be fruits and vegetables to reach your heart-protecting goal of at least five to nine servings a day. Blue blue-berry smoothies, hearty red marinara sauces, green salads, and multicolor vegetable soups should be your mainstays. Fruits and vegetables are not only a wonderful source of heart-helping phy-tonutrients but are also essentially devoid of saturated fat and have no cholesterol. Studies show that eating a diet high in fruit and vegetables may help to improve cholesterol levels, due in part to their unique phytonutrient mix as well as their abundance of fiber and lack of saturated fat and cholesterol.

You can buy fruits and vegetables to eat as snacks and side dishes, make vegetarian (meatless) main dishes, or add to poul-try stews or casseroles. You can also serve fresh fruit for dessert or freeze fruit (bananas, berries, melons, grapes) for a delicious fro-zen treat—such as a heart-healthy fresh dessert with low-fat yogurt topped with your favorite berries and a sprinkle of slivered almonds.

Display fresh fruit in a bowl in the kitchen to make it easier to grab as a snack, or wash and cut up raw vegetables (carrots, broccoli, cauliflower, lettuce, etc.) and store in the refrigerator for quick and easy use in cooking or snacking. To enjoy naturally healthy vegetables, season with herbs, spices, lemon juice, and balsamic vinegar.

In addition, frozen vegetables and fruits are an economical and convenient way to eat healthfully. Having a freezer stocked with these staples ensures you can whip up a delicious meal in minutes. Try frozen fruits such as blueberries, mixed berries, and cherries for the smoothies and fruit-based desserts you'll find in Chapter 9, or opt for frozen edamame (soybeans in their pods) for an easy appetizer for an Asian meal. Bagged, mixed veggies are perfect to make soups such as our Lentil and Mushroom Soup or salads such as our Black Bean Salad with Artichokes, Pepper, and Goat Cheese. Research shows that the nutrient content of frozen items is equal to or greater than that of fresh foods, which can lose many vitamins in the shipping and handling.

Breads, Cereals, and Other Whole Grains

When buying foods from the grains group, remember to choose whole-grain items. Whole-grain foods provide an abundance of fiber, minerals (such as magnesium), and phytonutrients to protect the heart; and they are lower on the glycemic index. They are also low in saturated fat and have no dietary cholesterol, with the exception of some bakery breads and sweet bread products made with whole milk, butter, and eggs.

Buy dry cereals but limit granola, muesli, and oat bran types that are made with coconut or coconut oil, which are high in saturated fat. Use fat-free or 1 percent milk, or try soy milk, almond milk, or rice milk instead of whole or low-fat (2 percent) milk to limit saturated fat and cholesterol.

Buy brown rice, and other whole grains (such as bulgur, quinoa, and kasha) to use as a healthy side dish. For a twist on pasta, try whole-wheat pasta and a hearty tomato-based sauce or a small amout of olive oil and garlic.

Avoid sweet baked goods that are made with lots of saturated fats and trans fats—mostly from butter, eggs, margarine, and whole milk—such as croissants, pastries, muffins, biscuits, butter rolls, and doughnuts. Try instead whole-grain healthy desserts (such as our Cinnamon Raisin Scones in Chapter 9), and other snacks that can be found in the natural foods aisle of your grocer or a health food store. Remember, though, that these should not be a staple—especially if you're trying to control your weight and cholesterol.

When shopping for grain products, don't forget to read the label to make sure the product includes "whole-grain" flours and has no "partially hydrogenated oil." Look for items such as these:

+ Whole-grain breads
+ Bread sticks made from whole grains or flatbreads
+ Ready-to-eat whole grain cereals without added sugar
+ Crackers made with whole grains
+ No-oil baked, whole-grain tortilla chips
+ Popcorn prepared at home with an air popper

Fats and Oils

Replacing saturated fats—such as those found primarily in meat and dairy products—with unsaturated fats—from plant-based sources—is a great way to protect your heart and keep your cholesterol in check. Just be sure to *be moderate in the amount of healthy fats or oils* to keep calories in check. When buying fats and oils, remember to choose liquid vegetable oils that are high in unsaturated fats such as canola, corn, olive, peanut, safflower, sesame, soybean, and sunflower oils.

Avoid butter, lard, and solid shortenings and avoid those containing partially hydrogenated oils. They are high in saturated fat, trans fats, and cholesterol. Also, buy light or nonfat mayonnaise. When choosing salad dressings, try making your own with olive oil and balsamic vinegar. Watch the portion to keep calories in check. For example, two tablespoons of regular Italian dressing can add as many as 14 grams of fat.

Margarine: Taking a Closer Look. We discussed the heart-harming effects of trans fats in Chapter 3. Unfortunately, these stealthy fats are sometimes difficult to spot. The harder the margarine or shortening, the more likely it is to contain more trans fat. Margarines that are free of trans fats are now available, and many contain cholesterol-cutting stanols. Read the ingredient label to choose margarine that is trans fat free or contains liquid vegetable oil rather than hydrogenated or partially hydrogenated oil as the first ingredient. Also, use the food label to choose margarine with the least amount of saturated fat. Choose soft tub or liquid margarine or vegetable oil spreads. Watch out for those partially hydrogenated oils.

Buyer Beware: What to Watch Out for at the Store

Beware of not-so-healthy "health" foods. Sports drinks and energy bars are not much more than sugar fortified with vitamins and minerals, each packing a whopping 200-plus calories per serving. The same goes for desserts and snack foods that are labeled "organic." These are no better than their "conventional" counterparts when it comes to nutrition.

Also, don't drown in the beverage aisle. Other than good old H_2O and calorie-free flavored waters, there's nothing in the beverage aisle you want to buy. This also goes for sugary, high-calorie iced teas, pseudosmoothies, sweetened milks, and coffee beverages. Don't be deterred by teas, though, as they provide a whole spectrum of antioxidant phytonutrients and help to reduce cholesterol.

Understanding Label Lingo

Deciphering labels can be a somewhat daunting task and one many people find intimidating. Armed with the knowledge in this book—including how to select whole grains and root out the bad fats—you'll be able to sleuth out the healthiest products for your heart. The very first thing you should do when deciding on a product is look at the ingredient list. This is the most detailed information on what a product contains and can help to answer the following questions.

❖ **Are the fats used in this product healthful or harmful?** Remember to look for foods made with olive, canola, or other healthful oils and avoid partially hydrogenated oils. This is of particular concern for packaged cereals, cookies, crackers, microwave popcorn, pastries, cake mixes, chips, and other cereal products, but it also applies to soups, frozen foods, and other premade convenience foods. Please refer to Chapter 3 to learn about your friends and foes of the fat world.

❖ **Is the product made with whole grains?** If the label does not say "whole," the product is made with refined flour. Instead of "wheat flour," for example, look for "whole wheat flour." This also applies for all other grains.

❖ **How much of each ingredient does the product contain?** The ingredient list is in descending order. The further down the list you go, the less of that ingredient the product contains.

❖ **Is the product full of sugar?** Avoid products with "high-fructose corn syrup" as well as fruit sweeteners appearing high on the ingredient list. Although sugars from fruits in nature may be more healthful when consumed in their natural state (i.e., as part of that Red Delicious apple), juice concentrate sweeteners have the same effect on blood sugar and the same number of calories as pure sugar.

❖ **How much of the product is a fruit or vegetable?** Although the product may be called "Strawberry Crunchies," after reading the food label you may find only a trace of strawberry flavor toward the end of the list. Choose foods that are nutrient-dense, and stay away from those that are merely empty calories.

Sizing It Up

Serving sizes are based on the amount of food people typically eat. However, many products contain multiple servings per package. Individual snack foods, for example, may contain 100 calories per "serving," but when you read the "number of servings" you find that energy bar you just ate contains three servings at 100 calories per serving, totaling 300 calories as opposed to the 100 you may have assumed. It doesn't just affect calories but also the amounts of all other nutritional components such as fat, sugar, and salt.

Use Table 7.1 as a guide to help you keep your portions and cholesterol under control.

Calories

Look at calories, and focus on where those calories come from. Use your calories as you would a daily stipend and try to make the most of each. Are your calories coming from healthy fats and whole grains, or are they derived from sugars and saturated and trans fats?

TABLE 7.1 **Serving Sizes**	
Food	**One Serving Size Equals ...**
Breads	1 slice bread or ½ bagel the size of a hockey puck
Rice, cooked	½ cup, which is the size of a cupcake wrapper
Pasta, cooked	½ cup, which is the size of an ice-cream scoop
Fruits and vegetables	1 piece the size of a tennis ball or ½ cup the size of a lightbulb
Meat, chicken, and fish	3 ounces lean meat, chicken, or fish, which is the size of a deck of cards or a checkbook
Dairy	1 ounce cheese, which is the size of about 4 dice
Fats, oils, and sweets	Use sparingly. A teaspoon of fat is about the size of the tip of your thumb.

The total fat panel provides the total amount of fat per serving and also breaks down the amount and type of each. Although trans fats may not yet be listed here on many products, you can decipher how much trans fat is in a product with a simple math equation.

By adding the saturated fat, monounsaturated fat, and polyunsaturated fat and then subtracting them from the total fat, you will determine the grams of trans fat in a specific product. For example, look at Smart Balance Popcorn. The total fat is 9 grams. The saturated fat is 3.5 grams, the monounsaturated fat is 2.5 grams, and the polyunsaturated fat is 3 grams.

9 − (3.5 grams saturated fat + 2.5 grams
monounsaturated fat + 3 grams polyunsaturated fat)
= 0 grams trans fat

Cholesterol

Dietary cholesterol can raise your blood cholesterol level, although usually not as much as saturated fat and trans fat can. The "daily values" section of the food label lists the amount of each nutrient in the food package based on current daily nutrition recommendations. Some labels list daily values for both 2,000- and 2,500-calorie diets.

Look at Label Claims

Another aspect of food labeling is label claims. Let's take a look at what some of the claims on your favorite foods mean.

A claim of "free" means that a food contains no amount (or a very small amount) of these nutrients: fat, saturated fat, cholesterol, sodium, sugar, and calories.

* "Calorie-free" = fewer than 5 calories per serving.
* "Fat-free" = fewer than 0.5 grams of fat per serving.

A claim of "low" can be used on all foods that can be eaten often without going over the limit for one or more of these nutrients: saturated fat, cholesterol, fat, sodium, and calories. Other words that mean "low" include *little, few,* and *low source of.*

* "Low saturated fat" = 1 gram or less per serving.
* "Low fat" = 3 grams or less per serving.
* "Low cholesterol" = 20 milligrams or less and 2 grams or less saturated fat per serving.

❖ "Low sodium" = 140 milligrams or less per serving.
❖ "Low calorie" = 40 calories or less per serving.

"Lean" and "extra lean" claims can be used to describe the saturated fat and fat content of meat, poultry, seafood, and game meats.

❖ "Lean" = fewer than 10 grams of fat and 4.5 grams or fewer of saturated fat, and fewer than 95 milligrams of cholesterol per serving.
❖ "Extra lean" = fewer than 5 grams of fat, fewer than 2 grams saturated fat, and fewer than 95 milligrams of cholesterol per serving.

Watching your serving size is still important. Just because something is "reduced fat" or "lighter" in calories does not give you carte blanche to load up! Base your meals around the fruits, vegetables, grains, and legumes we've described in Chapter 5, and prepare them a heart-healthy way for optimum benefit.

Dining Out for Heart Health

Dining out is full of palate pitfalls that can kick up your cholesterol more than a notch. Creamy sauces and added fats (many saturated and trans) are abundant. Here are a few tips to avoid dietary disasters when eating out.

❖ **Avoid fast foods.** This is a no-brainer. Eating deep-fried french fries cooked in partially hydrogenated oils (trans fats), a burger full of saturated fat, and a soda is a surefire way to fall off the cholesterol-cutting bandwagon. Many "healthy" fast-food establishments are also culprits, so ask for ingredients lists to make the wisest selection. If you must go, choose salads with grilled chicken, veggie burgers, or roasted turkey breast sandwiches and have the dressing served on the side so that you can control the amount.

✢ **Choose restaurants that have low-saturated-fat, low-cholesterol menu choices.** And, don't be afraid to make special requests—it's your right as a paying customer.

✢ **Control serving sizes.** Asking for a side-dish or appetizer-size serving, share a dish with a companion, or take some home.

✢ **Ask that gravy, butter, rich sauces, and salad dressing be served on the side.** That way, you can control the amount of saturated fat and cholesterol that you eat. A simple drizzle (not deluge!) of extra-virgin olive oil and balsamic vinegar can add lots of flavor.

✢ **Ask for substitutions.** Ask to substitute a salad or extra vegetables for chips, fries, coleslaw, or other extras—or just ask that the extras be left off of your plate.

✢ **Try a healthy alternative when ordering pizza.** Order vegetable toppings such as green pepper, onions, and mushrooms instead of meat or extra cheese. To make your pizza even lower in saturated fat, order it with half of the cheese or no cheese. Beware of the trans fats in commercially prepared pizzas; look in your grocer's freezer for organic, whole-grain pizza such as Amy's.

In addition, understanding how a food is prepared gives us important clues to its nutritional content. Table 7.2 provides the low–saturated fat, low-cholesterol cooking methods to look for when ordering as well as the terms to watch out for that indicate a dish is high in saturated fats and cholesterol.

The same menu clues that can be used when trying to pick the healthiest options at a restaurant can also be applied when figuring out the best methods to prepare heart-healthy meals at home. However, remember that when roasting, you should place meats on a rack so fat can drip away.

TABLE 7.2 Menu Clues: Cholesterol-Cutting Cooking Techniques	
Low–Saturated Fat/Cholesterol	**High–Saturated Fat/Cholesterol**
Steamed	In butter sauce
Cooked in its own juice (au jus)	Fried or crispy
Garden fresh	Creamed or in cream or cheese sauce
Broiled	Au gratin or *au fromage*
Baked	Escalloped
Roasted	Parmesan, hollandaise, or béarnaise
Poached	Marinated (in oil)
Cooked in tomato juice	Stewed or basted
Dry boiled (in wine or lemon juice)	Hash
Lightly sautéed	Casserole or pot pie
Lightly stir-fried	Pastry crust

Smart Substitutions

A few minor changes can make a big impact on your cholesterol levels. Let's take a look at some smart substitutions.

❖ Two tablespoons of butter can add an *extra* 16 grams of saturated fat and 22 grams of fat. However, one-quarter cup salsa has 0 grams of saturated fat and no cholesterol.

❖ Two tablespoons of regular creamy Italian salad dressing will add an *extra* 3 grams of saturated fat. Reduced-fat Italian dressing adds no saturated fat.

Planning Heart-Healthy Meals

Now that you know more about the foods you want to include and those you want to avoid for the healthiest heart, plus the best cooking methods to cut your cholesterol, Healing Gourmet offers suggestions that will help you to stick to your healthy eating plan when dining out or ordering in. A good rule of thumb is to avoid the bread basket. More often than not, the dough is made with unhealthy fats (hydrogenated margarine or butter) and refined grains. Flatbreads may be the healthiest option, but remember that filling up on bread adds unwanted calories with little nutritional benefit.

BREAKFAST
* ❖ Choose fresh fruit.
* ❖ Eat whole-grain bread or whole-wheat English muffin with peanut or almond butter or honey.
* ❖ Eat whole-grain cereal with low-fat (1 percent) or fat-free milk.
* ❖ Eat hot cereal (old-fashioned or steel-cut oats) with nonfat milk topped with fruit and a few pecans or walnuts.
* ❖ Have omelets with egg whites or egg substitute.
* ❖ Select whole-grain pancakes with fresh berries.
* ❖ Eat nonfat yogurt (and try adding cereal or fresh fruit).

BEVERAGES
* ❖ Drink water with lemon.
* ❖ Drink flavored sparkling water (noncaloric).

❖ Choose fat-free or low-fat (1 percent) milk.

❖ Try a juice spritzer (half fruit juice and half sparkling water).

❖ Drink tomato juice (reduced sodium).

❖ Drink tea (iced or hot, preferably green or black).

APPETIZERS

❖ Eat shrimp cocktail (but limit cocktail sauce—it's high in sodium).

❖ Have melons or fresh fruit.

❖ Select bean or broth-based soups.

❖ Eat salad with extra-virgin olive oil and vinegar or lemon juice.

❖ Have grilled vegetables.

❖ Have raw vegetables with low-fat dip or salsa.

❖ Eat vegetables with hummus or low-fat black bean dip.

ENTRÉES

❖ Poultry and fish are healthy choices when it comes to "meats."

❖ Select vegetarian dishes with whole grains, beans, and healthy sauces.

❖ Look for terms such as *baked, broiled, steamed, poached, lightly sautéed,* or *stir-fried,* and select those items.

❖ Ask for sauces and dressings on the side.

❖ Limit the amount of butter, margarine, and salt you use at the table.

SALADS/SALAD BARS

❖ Select fresh greens, lettuce, and spinach.

❖ Choose fresh vegetables—tomatoes, mushrooms, carrots, cucumbers, peppers, onion, radishes, and broccoli.

❖ Have beans, chickpeas, and kidney beans.

✢ Skip the nonvegetable choices—deli meats, bacon, egg, cheese, and croutons.

✢ Choose lower-calorie salad dressing or olive oil with lemon juice or vinegar.

Side Dishes

✢ Vegetables make the best additions to meals. Some restaurants are now offering healthier side dishes, such as sweet potato, whole-wheat pasta, and brown rice.

✢ Ask for side dishes without butter or margarine.

✢ Ask for mustard, salsa, or low-fat yogurt instead of sour cream or butter.

Dessert/Coffee

✢ Choose fresh fruit.

✢ Have sherbet or fruit sorbet. (These are usually fat-free and cholesterol-free.) Keep in mind, however, that these are high in sugar.

✢ Ask for low-fat milk for your coffee (instead of cream or half-and-half), and beware of coffee drinks that are full of calories, sugar, and fat. Better yet, try a cup of calorie-free, phytonutrient-rich tea with a lemon wedge or cinnamon.

Condiments

✢ Try horseradish.

✢ Have hot sauce.

✢ Try salsa.

✢ Have cocktail sauce (but limit your intake—it's high in sodium).

✢ Choose mustard.

✢ Have ketchup.

✢ Have vinegar.

✢ Eat lemon.

❖ Use herbs.
❖ Use spices.
❖ Try ginger.

You should already feel incredibly empowered by the information you have gained on the healing nutrients of certain foods. Now it's time to put all of this information to use in the delicious and healthy meal plans and recipes courtesy of Healing Gourmet. *Eat your medicine!*

8

My Daily Dose: Meal Plans to Get You Started

YOU DON'T HAVE to be a master chef to be a Healing Gourmet. Just let the principles and recipes in this book guide you. We have included recipes suited for the culinary novice, for those pressed for time, and for those who want to lose weight—and we do it without sacrificing any flavor. Mealtime should be one of the most enjoyable parts of your day, so let us help you to make it healthy!

In this chapter you will find seven-day meal plans for two different calorie levels: 1,500 calories and 2,000 calories. We recognize that readers will have different goals for their overall nutrition. The right calorie level for an individual is dependent upon his or her height, age, activity level, and goals for nutrition. Your registered dietitian can help you select an appropriate calorie level. However, no matter what your calorie level is, each of these levels includes the healthy principles of diet planning. All three menus use the following combination of sources:

* *Lean proteins* (ranging from 17 to 18 percent of total calories).
* *Healthy fats*—mostly monounsaturated and polyunsaturated fat (ranging from 30 to 35 percent of total calories).

✤ *Healthy carbohydrates* (ranging from 47 to 52 percent of total calories).

In addition, they all include foods that:

✤ Limit the use of saturated fat (to less than 8 percent of total calories)
✤ Avoid hydrogenated and partially hydrogenated fats (trans fats)
✤ Are low in cholesterol (fewer than 200 milligrams per day)
✤ Are moderate in sodium (most days fewer than 3,000 milligrams)
✤ Are high in fiber (minimum of 25 grams per day)

Finally, all these meals encourage:

✤ Eating a variety of foods
✤ Eating plenty of fruits and vegetables
✤ Using whole grains as the main choice for breads, cereals, crackers, and pasta
✤ Using whole foods, free-range poultry, fish, and fresh herbs and spices

And, most important, they taste great!

In the menus in this chapter, you'll find meals for breakfast, lunch, and dinner, as well as snacks to eat throughout the day. We also include information about the nutritional content for the day and feature recipes from Chapter 9, which are indicated with an asterisk (*). We have also included a "veg out" option, which features a vegetarian alternative for dinner. Non-meat eaters can also find more vegetarian alternatives to the meat-filled lunches in the Soups and Salads section in our recipe chapter. Please note that if you select the veg out option, the calories and other nutrients (proteins, fats, carbohydrates, etc.) will vary somewhat from the information given in the meal plan. In addition, we recommend drinking six to eight glasses of water a day. You can substitute low-sodium sparkling water for two of the six glasses a day and spring water with a lemon wedge to add some variety.

My Meal Plans: 1,500 Calories

If you are overweight, achieving a healthy weight will help to prevent heart disease and reduce cholesterol. Always talk with your doctor or registered dietitian to decide what is right for you.

Day 1

BREAKFAST
¾ cup high-fiber cereal topped with
¾ cup blueberries,
1 ounce almonds, and
¾ cup 1 percent milk
Spring water

LUNCH
2 slices whole-wheat bread topped with
1 ounce low-fat mozzarella cheese,
2½ ounces turkey breast,
2 slices tomatoes, and
1 teaspoon yellow mustard

SNACK
1 apple
1 tablespoon almond butter

DINNER
1 serving Grilled Chicken with Chile-Lime Sauce*
½ cup snap beans and
½ cup broccoli stir-fried in
½ tablespoon olive oil
1 sweet potato

Veg Out! *Substitute Black Bean Burritos for the chicken dish if you like.*

SNACK
½ cup plain nonfat yogurt topped with
½ cup strawberries

What's inside? 1,512 calories, 95 grams protein, 197 grams carbohydrates, 55 grams total fat, 152 milligrams cholesterol, 11.5 grams saturated fat, 1,215 milligrams sodium, 46 grams dietary fiber

---

Day 2

BREAKFAST
Omelet made with ½ cup egg substitute,
2 slices white onion, and
¼ cup chopped green bell pepper cooked in
2 teaspoons canola oil
1 slice toasted whole-wheat bread topped with
1 teaspoon creamy peanut butter
1 orange

LUNCH
2 ounces roasted chicken
1 cup mixed greens salad topped with
1 tablespoon balsamic vinaigrette

2 whole-wheat breadsticks
1 cup skim milk
1 peach

SNACK
1 ounce almonds
Herbal tea

DINNER
1 serving Turkey Bolognese*
Cucumber and cherry tomato salad topped with
1 tablespoon oil and vinegar dressing

Veg Out! *Try our N'Orleans Red Beans and Rice for a vegetarian alternative to the turkey dish.*

SNACK
½ cup nonfat vanilla frozen yogurt

What's inside? 1,483 calories, 84.5 grams protein, 178 grams carbohydrates, 52 grams total fat, 124 milligrams cholesterol, 11 grams saturated fat, 978 milligrams sodium, 24 grams dietary fiber

---

Day 3

BREAKFAST
¾ cup bran flakes cereal topped with
½ cup fresh strawberries and
½ cup skim milk
1 whole-wheat English muffin topped with
1 tablespoon almond butter

LUNCH
1 ounce whole-wheat pita topped with
2 ounces turkey breast,
½ cup fresh alfalfa sprouts,
3 slices tomato, and
2 teaspoons yellow mustard
1 cup pineapple
½ cup skim milk

SNACK
1 cup baby carrots
2 tablespoons hummus

DINNER
1 serving Broiled Mahimahi with Red Bell Pepper Sauce*
Spring water

Veg Out! *Try our Black Bean Burritos for a protein-rich vegetarian dish.*

SNACK
1 banana
Herbal tea

What's inside? 1,513 calories, 82 grams protein, 194 grams carbohydrate, 56 grams total fat, 129 milligrams cholesterol, 10 grams saturated fat, 1,996 milligrams sodium, 28 grams dietary fiber

---

Day 4

BREAKFAST
1 whole-wheat bagel topped with
1 tablespoon low-fat cream cheese
½ cup orange juice

LUNCH
½ cup garbanzo beans combined with
½ cup yellow corn,
2 slices fresh avocado,
1½ cups mixed green salad,
2 teaspoons olive oil, and
1 tablespoon vinegar
1 whole-wheat dinner roll
1 cup skim milk

SNACK
1 ounce mixed nuts

DINNER
1 serving Fajita Burgers*
Romaine lettuce with carrots and tomatoes topped with
1 tablespoon balsamic vinaigrette
Spring water

SNACK
1 cup watermelon
Herbal tea

What's inside? 1,492 calories, 65 grams protein, 205 grams
carbohydrates, 55 grams total fat, 23 milligrams cholesterol, 11 grams
saturated fat, 1,415 milligrams sodium, 39 grams dietary fiber

---

Day 5

BREAKFAST
1 whole-grain waffle topped with
1 cup raspberries,
1 tablespoon almond butter, and

2 teaspoons maple syrup
Spring water

MIDMORNING SNACK
½ cup broccoli florets
3 tablespoons hummus
1 cup decaffeinated green tea

LUNCH
2 slices whole-wheat bread topped with
1 ounce fat-free Swiss cheese,
2 ounces low-salt, low-fat ham,
2 teaspoons yellow mustard,
3 slices tomato, and
2 leaves butterhead lettuce
1 medium kiwi fruit
½ cup skim milk

SNACK
1 cup strawberry low-fat yogurt

DINNER
1 serving Roasted Red Pepper and Pesto Sandwich*
½ cup skim milk
Spring water

SNACK
1 apple
Decaffeinated green tea with lemon

What's inside? 1,491 calories, 71 grams protein, 196 grams carbohydrates, 52 grams total fat, 78 milligrams cholesterol, 13 grams saturated fat, 2,934 milligrams sodium, 29 grams dietary fiber

---

Day 6

BREAKFAST
¾ cup old-fashioned oatmeal
½ medium apple
1 slice whole-wheat toast topped with
2 teaspoons peanut butter
1 cup skim milk

LUNCH
2 slices rye bread topped with
3 ounces sardines,
2 teaspoons yellow mustard, and
2 slices tomato
1 grapefruit
Spring water

SNACK
1 ounce hazelnuts
Herbal tea

DINNER
1 serving Shanghai Chicken Kabobs*
1 cup mixed green salad topped with
1 tablespoon balsamic vinaigrette
Spring water

Veg Out! *Enjoy our Roasted Italian Vegetable Terrine.*

SNACK
¾ cup vanilla low-fat frozen yogurt topped with
½ cup fresh strawberries
Herbal tea

What's inside? 1,490 calories, 88 grams protein, 171 grams
carbohydrates, 51 grams total fat, 206 milligrams cholesterol, 8 grams
saturated fat, 206 milligrams sodium, 21 grams dietary fiber

Day 7

BREAKFAST
¾ cup shredded wheat topped with
1 banana and
½ cup skim milk
Spring water

MIDMORNING SNACK
1 pear
1 cup decaffeinated green tea

LUNCH
3 ounces grilled chicken
2 whole-wheat crackers
2 cups salad combined with
½ cup chopped carrots,
Cucumber slices,
1 tablespoon extra-virgin olive oil, and
1 tablespoon balsamic vinegar
Spring water

SNACK
1 ounce peanuts
Herbal tea

DINNER
1 serving Old-Fashioned Chicken Stew*
½ cup broccoli,

½ cup red peppers, and
½ cup onions stir-fried in
1 tablespoon olive oil
1 whole-wheat dinner roll
Spring water

Veg Out! *Enjoy Zucchini Lasagna as an alternative to the chicken.*

SNACK
½ whole-wheat English muffin topped with
1 tablespoon peanut butter
Herbal tea

What's inside? 1,519 calories, 79 grams protein, 179 grams carbohydrates, 61 grams total fat, 86 milligrams cholesterol, 10 grams saturated fat, 1,673 milligrams sodium, 32 grams dietary fiber

---

My Meal Plans: 2,000 Calories

These meal plans are suitable for most people looking to maintain a healthy weight. However, your age, your metabolism, your exercise habits, and other factors also come into play. So once again, we emphasize the importance of talking with your doctor to find a plan that's right for you.

Day 1

BREAKFAST
1 whole-wheat English muffin
Omelet made with 2 egg whites,
¼ cup fresh mushrooms, and
¼ cup chopped green bell peppers cooked in

½ tablespoon canola oil
1 cup low-fat strawberry yogurt
1 tangerine

MIDMORNING SNACK
¼ cup hummus
10 baby carrots
1 cup decaffeinated green tea

LUNCH
1 cup lentil soup
3 ounces salmon
2 cups mixed greens salad
½ cup cantaloupe
1 cup skim milk

SNACK
2 ounces trail mix
Herbal tea

DINNER
1 serving Sole Florentine*
Spring water

Veg Out! *Substitute Black Bean Burritos for the fish dish if you like.*

SNACK
4 crispbread rye crackers topped with
2 tablespoons all-natural peanut butter

What's inside? 2,014 calories, 127 grams protein, 235 grams
carbohydrates, 70 grams total fat, 170 milligrams cholesterol, 14 grams
saturated fat, 2,899 milligrams sodium, 37 grams dietary fiber

---

Day 2

BREAKFAST
1 cup Wheatena hot cereal topped with
1 ounce pecans and
1 cup skim milk
1 banana

LUNCH
2 slices whole-wheat bread topped with
4 ounces tuna (in water),
3 slices tomato,
2 lettuce leaves, and
2 tablespoons soy mayonnaise
1 cup low-fat milk
Spring water

SNACK
1 apple topped with
2 tablespoons almond butter
Herbal tea

DINNER
1 serving Black Bean Burritos*
Spring water

SNACK
1 cup chocolate low-fat frozen yogurt
½ ounce walnuts

What's inside? 2,010 calories, 97 grams protein, 243 grams carbohydrates, 79 grams total fat, 63 milligrams cholesterol, 13 grams saturated fat, 2,286 milligrams sodium, 41 grams dietary fiber

Day 3

BREAKFAST
1 whole-grain bagel topped with
1 tablespoon low-fat cream cheese
½ cup orange juice
1 cup low-fat blueberry yogurt

LUNCH
3 ounces skinless chicken breast
2 cups tossed green salad combined with
3 ounces marinated artichoke hearts,
5 cherry tomatoes,
8 mushrooms,
1 tablespoon extra-virgin olive oil, and
1 tablespoon balsamic vinegar
1 cup melon
1 whole-wheat roll
1 cup skim milk

SNACK
1 ounce sunflower seeds

DINNER
1 serving Turkey Stuffed Cabbage*
Cucumber salad with cherry tomatoes and
1 tablespoon balsamic vinegar salad dressing
1 cup pineapple
Spring water

Veg Out! *Try our Fajita Burgers as an alternative.*

Snack
1 ounce peanuts
Herbal tea

What's inside? 1,969 calories, 110 grams protein, 247 grams carbohydrates, 68 grams total fat, 168 milligrams cholesterol, 13 grams saturated fat, 2,041 milligrams sodium, 35 grams dietary fiber

---

Day 4

Breakfast
1 cup shredded wheat topped with
2 tablespoons raisins and
1 cup skim milk
2 slices whole-wheat toast topped with
1½ tablespoons all-natural peanut butter

Midmorning Snack
1 cup decaffeinated green tea
1 cup strawberries

Lunch
1 cup minestrone soup, unsalted
¾ cup tabbouleh
¼ cup avocado
1 whole-wheat roll
1 orange

Snack
1 cup low-fat strawberry yogurt
Low-sodium sparkling water

DINNER
1 serving Quick Chicken Creole*
Salad made with 1 cup romaine lettuce,
4 slices tomato, and
1 tablespoon vinegar and oil salad dressing
1 kiwi fruit

Veg Out! *Our Caribbean Black Beans and Rice is a delicious veggie alternative.*

SNACK
1 ounce pistachio nuts
Herbal tea

What's inside? 2,038 calories, 85 grams protein, 280 grams carbohydrates, 78 grams total fat, 82 milligrams cholesterol, 14 grams saturated fat, 2,002 milligrams sodium, 45 grams dietary fiber

---

Day 5

BREAKFAST
2 whole-wheat frozen waffles topped with
2 tablespoons almond butter and
1 tablespoon maple syrup
1 cup blueberries
Spring water

LUNCH
2 slices rye bread topped with
3 ounces turkey breast,
1 tablespoon heart-healthy mayonnaise,
2 leaves butterhead lettuce, and

3 slices tomato
1 pear
1 cup skim milk

SNACK
1 ounce peanuts

DINNER
1 serving Trout Veracruz*
⅔ cup quinoa
1 cup mixed greens salad with
Cucumber slices and topped with
1 tablespoon vinegar and oil dressing
1 apple
Spring water

Veg Out! *Try our Roasted Red Pepper and Pesto Sandwich paired up with a mixed greens salad as an alternative.*

SNACK
1 cup nonfat lemon yogurt
1 cup decaffeinated green tea

What's inside? 2,023 calories, 107 grams protein, 256 grams carbohydrates, 71 grams total fat, 279 milligrams cholesterol, 12 grams saturated fat, 1,437 milligrams sodium, 25 grams dietary fiber

---

Day 6

BREAKFAST
1 cup Raisin Bran cereal topped with
1 banana and

1 cup skim milk
1 serving egg substitute cooked in
½ tablespoon canola oil

Lunch
1 cup vegetarian stew
1 whole-wheat pita topped with
1 ounce crabmeat
1 cup grapes

Snack
1 tablespoon all-natural peanut butter
1 apple

Dinner
2 slices Portobello Pizza*
1 cup mixed greens salad combined with
5 green olives,
4 tomato wedges,
2 slices red onion,
1 tablespoon extra-virgin olive oil, and
1 tablespoon vinegar
Spring water

Snack
1 ounce almonds
Herbal tea

What's inside? 2,012 calories, 125 grams protein, 235 grams carbohydrates, 71 grams total fat, 78 milligrams cholesterol, 14 grams saturated fat, 2,891 milligrams sodium, 33 grams dietary fiber

---

Day 7

BREAKFAST
1 cup old-fashioned oatmeal topped with
2 tablespoons walnuts and
1 tablespoon dried cranberries
1 orange
⅓ cup low-fat cottage cheese

MIDMORNING SNACK
1 cup nonfat plain yogurt topped with
½ cup strawberries
1 cup decaffeinated green tea

LUNCH
1 whole-wheat tortilla topped with
½ cup vegetarian refried beans,
1 ounce low-fat Monterey Jack cheese, and
½ cup salsa
1 nectarine
Spring water

SNACK
1 ounce mixed nuts

DINNER
1 serving Oven-Fried Catfish*
1 sweet potato
½ cup onions,
½ cup zucchini, and
½ cup red bell pepper stir-fried in
1 tablespoon olive oil

1 whole-wheat roll
1 cup cantaloupe
Spring water

Veg Out! *Try our Garden Fresh Pasta Sauce served with whole-wheat linguine and a mixed green salad as an alternative.*

SNACK
1 whole-wheat English muffin topped with
2 tablespoons peanut butter
½ cup skim milk

What's inside? 2,025 calories, 104 grams protein, 257 grams carbohydrates, 78 grams total fat, 98 milligrams cholesterol, 15 grams saturated fat, 2,830 milligrams sodium, 43 grams dietary fiber

---

Gourmet Rx:
The Recipes

Now that we've explored the nutrients and foods to help you lower cholesterol and protect against heart disease, let's put it together with these delicious meals. Here you'll find fifty recipes, suited for the novice chef, that deliver a healthy dose of nutrients and flavor. Please note that optional ingredients are not included in the nutritional information. Bon appétit!

Soups and Salads

No longer revered as side items, soups and salads take a starring role in your health. Fresh vegetables and a variety of beans help protect your cells from oxidative damage.

Mediterranean Fish Chowder

Take your taste buds on a trip to the Mediterranean with this delicious chowder. It's no wonder the Mediterraneans enjoy less heart disease. This tomato-based chowder delivers heart-healthy lycopene and omega-3 fatty acids.

> 2 tablespoons extra-virgin olive oil
> 1 large clove garlic, minced
> 3 large carrots, cut in thin strips
> 2 cups sliced celery
> ½ cup chopped yellow onion
> ¼ cup chopped green bell pepper
> 1 28-ounce can whole tomatoes, cut up, with liquid
> 1 cup clam juice
> ¼ teaspoon crushed dried thyme
> ¼ teaspoon crushed dried basil
> ⅛ teaspoon black pepper
> 2 pounds varied fish fillets (haddock, perch, flounder, cod, sole, and so forth), cut into 1-inch-square cubes
> ¼ cup minced fresh Italian flat-leaf parsley

Heat oil in large sauce pan. Sauté garlic, carrots, celery, onion, and green pepper in oil for 3 minutes. Add tomatoes, clam juice, thyme, basil, and pepper. Cover and simmer for 10 to 15 minutes or until vegetables are fork tender. Add fish and parsley. Simmer, covered, for 5 to 10 minutes more or until fish flakes easily when tested with a fork and is opaque. Serve hot.

Serves 8 (serving size: 1 cup)

Servings of fruits and vegetables: 1 vegetable; **cholesterol-lowering phytonutrients:** sulfides, carotenoids, lycopene

Nutrition information: 174 calories, 23 grams protein, 5 grams total fat, 1 gram saturated fat, no trans fat, 55 milligrams cholesterol, 9 grams carbohydrates, 2 grams dietary fiber, 340 milligrams sodium

Corn Chowder

This creamy and comforting soup provides a bevy of B vitamins.

1 tablespoon vegetable oil
2 tablespoons finely diced celery
2 tablespoons finely diced yellow onion
2 tablespoons finely diced green bell pepper
1 10-ounce package frozen whole-kernel corn
1 cup peeled, ½-inch-diced raw potatoes
¼ teaspoon salt
Freshly ground black pepper
¼ teaspoon sweet paprika
2 cups low-fat (1 percent) or skim milk
2 tablespoons flour
2 tablespoons chopped fresh Italian flat-leaf parsley

Heat oil in medium saucepan. Add celery, onion, and green pepper and sauté for 2 minutes. Add corn, potatoes, 1 cup water, salt, pepper, and paprika. Bring to a boil; reduce heat to medium and cook, covered, for about 10 minutes or until potatoes are tender. Place ½ cup milk in a jar with tight-fitting lid. Add flour and shake vigorously. (Alternately, whisk in a large measuring cup or small bowl to blend.) Add gradually to cooked vegetables, and add remaining milk. Cook, stirring constantly, until mixture comes to a boil and thickens. Serve garnished with parsley.

Serves 8 (serving size: 1 cup)

Servings of fruits and vegetables: 1 vegetable; **cholesterol-lowering phytonutrients:** lutein, sulfides, carotenoids

---

Nutrition information: 100 calories, 4 grams protein, 2.5 grams total fat, 0.5 gram saturated fat, 0.02 gram trans fat, 5 milligrams cholesterol, 16 grams carbohydrates, 1.5 grams dietary fiber, 105 milligrams sodium

---

Middle Eastern Bulgur Salad

A nutritious staple in the Middle East, bulgur wheat consists of wheat kernels that have been steamed, dried, and crushed. It has a tender, chewy texture and is perfect for a light lunch or as an accompaniment to a light fish or chicken dish.

 1 tablespoon extra-virgin olive oil
 1 cup diced Vidalia or other sweet yellow onion
 2 large cloves garlic, minced
 1 cup bulgur

1 15½-ounce can whole tomatoes
⅓ cup fresh Italian flat-leaf parsley or basil
Freshly ground black pepper

In medium saucepan, heat oil. Add onion and stir with a wooden spoon 1 minute. Stir in garlic and bulgur; cook for 2 minutes. Add tomatoes, 1¾ cups water, and parsley or basil. Reduce heat, cover, and simmer for 15 to 20 minutes. Fluff with a fork and serve. Top with freshly ground black pepper.

Serves 6 (serving size: 1 cup)

Servings of fruits and vegetables: ⅓ vegetable; **cholesterol-lowering phytonutrients:** sulfides, carotenoids, lycopene, allicin

Nutrition information: 140 calories, 4.5 grams protein, 3 grams total fat, no saturated fat, no trans fat, no cholesterol, 27 grams carbohydrates, 4 grams dietary fiber, 200 milligrams sodium

Carrot Ginger Bisque

If you've never experienced fresh gingerroot, its flavor is peppery and slightly sweet—the perfect complement to carrots in this delightful bisque.

2 pounds carrots, washed and chopped
1 large gingerroot, peeled and sliced thin
2 tablespoons canola oil
2 cups soy milk or skim milk
½ teaspoon freshly ground nutmeg
Freshly ground black pepper (optional)

Fill a large pot with water. Add carrots, half of the ginger, and oil. Bring to a boil and cook until carrots are tender. Drain carrots, reserving 2 cups of the broth. Put carrots and broth into a food processor. Process in batches until smooth, adding the milk and additional water to desired consistency. Return mixture to pot to keep warm; serve with a sprinkle of nutmeg and freshly ground black pepper, if desired.

Serves 8 (serving size: 1 cup)

Servings of fruits and vegetables: 2 vegetables; **cholesterol-lowering phytonutrients:** gingerols, carotenoids, phytoestrogens

Nutrition information: 120 calories, 4 grams protein, 5 grams total fat, 0.5 gram saturated fat, no trans fat, no cholesterol, 16 grams carbohydrates, 4 grams dietary fiber, 115 milligrams sodium

---

*W*ild Rice Salad

Luxurious flavor and nutty crunch make wild rice the perfect grain to add to this colorful, flavor-filled salad.

4 cups wild rice, cooked or soaked overnight
2 medium cucumbers, chopped fine
2 medium red or yellow bell peppers, chopped fine
1 small jicama, shredded
2 medium tomatoes, chopped fine
4 celery stalks, chopped fine
6 scallions or 1 small yellow onion, chopped fine

1 cup chopped fresh cilantro, Italian flat-leaf parsley,
  or basil
1 large avocado, peeled and pitted
½ to 1 cup tomatillo juice or sauerkraut juice
Pinch of cayenne
Chopped cilantro, basil, or parsley to taste

Put first eight ingredients into a large bowl and toss together.
In a separate bowl, mix together the next four ingredients until
creamy. Drizzle dressing over salad and serve.

Serves 8 (serving size: 1 cup)

Servings of fruits and vegetables: ½ fruit, 3 vegetables; **cholesterol-lowering phytonutrients:** sulfides, carotenoids, lycopene

Nutrition information: 186 calories, 6 grams protein, 4 grams total fat,
0.6 gram saturated fat, no cholesterol, no trans fat, 33 grams
carbohydrates, 8 grams dietary fiber, 34 milligrams sodium

Marinated Provençale Salad

*Garlic, tomatoes, and olive oil are major trademarks of dishes from
the Provençe region in the southeastern part of France.*

4 large red bell peppers, quartered lengthwise
4 medium yellow zucchini, sliced thin lengthwise
3 tablespoons extra-virgin olive oil
4 large Japanese eggplants, sliced lengthwise
¼ cup minced fresh basil

¼ cup minced fresh herbs (or any blend of oregano, marjoram, thyme, parsley)
3 large cloves garlic, pressed
½ cup balsamic vinegar
6 tomatoes, sliced
¼ cup Nicoise olives

Preheat broiler; place peppers skin side up on baking sheet.
Broil until skin blackens, rearranging as needed. Place in a paper
bag and set aside to cool and soften. Arrange zucchini on baking
sheet, brush with oil, and broil for 4 minutes on each side. Repeat
with eggplants; keep veggies separate. Peel and thinly slice peppers. Mix all herbs and garlic in bowl. Alternate layers of zucchini,
pepper strips, and eggplants in a casserole dish with a tight fitting
lid, drizzling with oil, vinegar, and herb mixture between each
layer. Save leftover oil, vinegar, and herbs. Chill overnight. When
ready to serve, arrange tomato slices atop vegetables. Drizzle with
remaining oil, vinegar, and herbs. Top with olives, and serve.

Serves 8 (serving size: 1 cup)

Servings of fruits and vegetables: 10 vegetables; **cholesterol-lowering
phytonutrients:** lutein, sulfides, carotenoids, lycopene

Nutrition information: 190 calories, 5.5 grams protein, 7 grams total
fat, 1 gram saturated fat, no trans fat, no cholesterol, 34 grams
carbohydrates, 13 grams dietary fiber, 160 milligrams sodium

*L*entil and Mushroom Soup

Don't limit yourself to the traditional dried brown lentils—try red or yellow lentils for a change of color and taste.

1 tablespoon extra-virgin olive oil
2 cups chopped yellow onion
2 large cloves garlic, minced
2 cups lentils, rinsed
2 cups diced carrots
2 cups sliced mushrooms
1 cup diced celery
1 bay leaf
1 teaspoon rosemary
Pinch crushed red pepper
1 cup chopped and seeded plum tomatoes
1 tablespoon red wine vinegar
½ cup fresh Italian flat-leaf parsley

Heat oil in saucepan. Add onion, and sauté until softened, about 10 minutes. Add garlic; stir. Add 6 cups water, lentils, carrots, mushrooms, celery, bay leaf, rosemary, and crushed red pepper. Bring to a boil, reduce heat to medium, and simmer for 45 minutes. Discard bay leaf. Add tomatoes and vinegar, and simmer for 5 minutes. Sprinkle with parsley, and serve.

Serves 6 (serving size: 1 cup)

Servings of fruits and vegetables: 2½ vegetables; **cholesterol-lowering phytonutrients:** phytoestrogens, allicin, sulfides, lycopene

Nutrition information: 310 calories, 21 grams protein, 2.5 grams total fat, no saturated fat, no trans fat, no cholesterol, 55 grams carbohydrates, 11 grams dietary fiber, 55 milligrams sodium

Black Bean Salad with Artichokes, Pepper, and Goat Cheese

*This salad boasts low-GI, high-fiber black beans to help reduce cho-
lesterol, plus lycopene and vitamins for a healthy heart. Rinse the marinated artichoke hearts to help reduce the amount of fat.*

1 16-ounce can black beans
⅔ cup chopped red bell pepper
½ cup Vidalia or other yellow onion
1 6-ounce jar marinated artichoke hearts, chopped
1 bunch fresh arugula, stemmed, rinsed, and drained
2 ounces soft mild goat cheese (Montrachet)

Combine beans, bell pepper, and onion in medium bowl. Stir
in artichokes. Layer arugula on two plates. Spoon bean salad over
arugula. Top with goat cheese, and serve.

Serves 2 (serving size: half of recipe)

Servings of fruits and vegetables: 3 vegetables; **cholesterol-lowering
phytonutrients:** phytoestrogens, carotenoids, sulfides

Nutrition information: 380 calories, 22 grams protein, 13 grams total
fat, 4 grams saturated fat, no trans fat, 15 milligrams cholesterol, 47
grams carbohydrates, 17 grams dietary fiber, 1,130 milligrams sodium

Greek Orzo and Shrimp Salad

Protein-rich shrimp and orzo—a tiny, rice-shaped pasta perfect for salads—get accompanied with herbs and vegetables for a dish to reel in.

2 cups orzo
4 scallions, chopped
½ cup crumbled feta cheese
2 tablespoons chopped fresh dill, plus sprigs
2 tablespoons fresh lemon juice
1 pound shrimp, peeled and deveined
1 medium cucumber, quartered lengthwise and chopped
1 pint cherry tomatoes, halved

Cook orzo until tender, for about 10 minutes; drain and rinse. Drain again. Place orzo in a large bowl. Add scallions, feta, dill, and lemon juice. Cook shrimp in boiling water for about 2 minutes or just until white and done, being careful not to overcook; drain and rinse. Stir into orzo mixture. Add cucumber and tomatoes. Garnish with dill sprigs, and serve.

Serves 4 (serving size: 1 cup)

Servings of fruits and vegetables: approximately 2½ vegetables; **cholesterol-lowering phytonutrients:** sulfides, lycopene, terpenes

Nutrition information: 370 calories, 30 grams protein, 6 grams total fat, 3.5 grams saturated fat, no trans fat, 185 milligrams cholesterol, 50 grams carbohydrates, 4 grams dietary fiber, 420 milligrams sodium

Texas Chili

Texans have a big taste for chili . . . and this recipe would please any of 'em (no matter where they live!). Full of flavor, fiber, and phytonutrients this chili may help you get a harness on your cholesterol.

2 teaspoons canola oil
½ cup chopped yellow onion
½ cup chopped green bell pepper
1 clove garlic, chopped
1 small jalapeño pepper, seeded and minced (or ½ teaspoon cayenne pepper)
1 teaspoon ground cumin
1 14½-ounce can tomatoes, diced or broken up, with liquid
1 teaspoon minced fresh oregano
1 tablespoon chopped cilantro
1 15-ounce can pinto beans, rinsed and drained (or 2 cups cooked beans)
Freshly ground black pepper

In a medium saucepan, heat oil over medium-high heat. Sauté onion, bell pepper, and garlic until onions are soft, about 6 to 7 minutes. Mix in jalapeño and cumin and cook, stirring constantly, until cumin is fragrant, about 30 seconds. Add tomatoes, oregano, and cilantro; reduce heat to medium; and simmer for 10 minutes or until mixture thickens slightly. Add beans, and add pepper to taste. Simmer gently for 10 minutes. Let sit for 20 minutes to allow flavors to blend.

Serves 8 (serving size: 1 cup)

Servings of fruits and vegetables: approximately 2½ vegetables; **cholesterol-lowering phytonutrients:** phytoestrogens, lycopene, sulfides

Nutrition information: 340 calories, 17 grams protein, 6 grams total fat, 0.5 gram saturated fat, no trans fat, 15 milligrams cholesterol, 60 grams carbohydrates, 2 grams dietary fiber, 570 milligrams sodium

Chicken and Poultry

Poultry provides a bevy of B vitamins that help reduce levels of heart-harming homocysteine while delivering a good source of blood sugar–balancing protein.

*A*rroz con Pollo

Literally translated "rice with chicken," this tasty Spanish and Mexican dish is always a hit and provides cholesterol-crushing veggies.

6 chicken pieces (legs and breasts), skinned
2 teaspoons vegetable oil
2 medium tomatoes, seeded and chopped
½ cup chopped green bell pepper
¼ cup chopped red bell pepper
¼ cup diced celery
1 medium carrot, grated
¼ cup frozen corn
½ cup chopped yellow onion
¼ cup chopped fresh cilantro
2 large cloves garlic, chopped fine
⅛ teaspoon salt
⅛ teaspoon black pepper
2 cups uncooked, long-grain rice
½ cup frozen peas
2 ounces Spanish olives, pitted
¼ cup raisins

In a large pot, brown chicken pieces in oil. Add 4 cups water, tomatoes, green and red peppers, celery, carrot, corn, onion, cilantro, garlic, salt, and black pepper. Cover and cook over medium heat for 20 to 30 minutes or until chicken is cooked through. Remove chicken from the pot and place in the refrigerator. Add rice, peas, and olives to the pot. Cover pot and cook over low heat for about 20 minutes until rice is cooked. Cut chicken into pieces, then return to the pot adding raisins; cook for another 8 minutes.

Serves 6 (serving size: 1 cup rice and 1 piece chicken)

Servings of fruits and vegetables: 1/3 fruit, approximately 1 1/2 vegetables; **cholesterol-lowering phytonutrients:** lutein, sulfides, carotenoids

Nutrition information: 480 calories, 33 grams protein, 9 grams total fat, 2 grams saturated fat, no trans fat, 75 milligrams cholesterol, 64 grams carbohydrates, 5 grams dietary fiber, 300 milligrams sodium

Turkey Bolognese

Turkey gives a new twist to this dish named after the rich cookery style of Bologna, Italy. Our version uses lean ground turkey to help you protect your heart and reduce cholesterol.

Nonstick cooking spray
1 pound 98 percent lean ground turkey
1 28-ounce can tomatoes, cut up
1 cup finely chopped green bell pepper
1 cup finely chopped yellow onion

2 cloves garlic, minced
1 teaspoon crushed dried oregano
1 teaspoon black pepper
1 pound spaghetti, uncooked

Spray a large skillet with nonstick spray coating. Preheat over medium-high heat. Add turkey and cook, stirring occasionally, for 5 minutes. Drain any fat and discard. Stir tomatoes with their juice, green pepper, onion, garlic, oregano, and black pepper into the turkey. Bring to a boil; reduce heat. Simmer covered for 15 minutes, stirring occasionally. Remove cover; simmer for 15 additional minutes. (If you'd prefer a creamier sauce, give sauce a whirl in your blender or food processor.) Meanwhile, cook spaghetti in a large pot of unsalted boiling water for 10 to 12 minutes. Drain well. Serve sauce over spaghetti.

Serves 6 (serving size: ½ cup sauce and 1 cup spaghetti)

Servings of fruits and vegetables: approximately ½ vegetable; **cholesterol-lowering phytonutrients:** sulfides, lycopene

Nutrition information: 460 calories, 27 grams protein, 9 grams total fat, 2 grams saturated fat, no trans fat, 55 milligrams cholesterol, 67 grams carbohydrates, 4 grams dietary fiber, 260 milligrams sodium

Turkey Stuffed Cabbage

A hearty European entrée, this savory dish is full of fiber and heart-helping phytonutrients.

1 head green cabbage
1 pound 98 percent lean ground turkey

2 small yellow onions, 1 minced and 1 sliced
1 slice stale whole-wheat bread, crumbled
1 tablespoon fresh lemon juice
⅛ teaspoon black pepper
1 16-ounce can diced tomatoes
1 medium carrot, sliced

Rinse and core cabbage. Carefully remove ten outer leaves, place them in saucepan, and cover with boiling water. Simmer for 10 minutes. Remove cooked cabbage leaves and drain on paper toweling. Shred ½ cup of raw cabbage and set aside. Brown ground turkey and minced onion in skillet. Drain and discard any fat. Place cooked and drained meat mixture, bread crumbs, ¼ cup water, lemon juice, and pepper in mixing bowl.

Drain tomatoes, reserving liquid, and add ½ cup tomato juice from can to meat mixture. Mix well, and then place ¼ cup filling on each parboiled, drained cabbage leaf. Place folded side down in skillet. Add tomatoes, sliced onion, 1 cup water, shredded cabbage, and carrot. Cover and simmer for about 30 minutes (or until cabbage is tender), basting occasionally. Remove cabbage rolls to serving platter; serve warm.

Serves 5 (serving size: 2 rolls)

Servings of fruits and vegetables: 4 vegetables; **cholesterol-lowering phytonutrients:** lutein, sulfides, carotenoids

---

Nutrition information: 260 calories, 22 grams protein, 9 grams total fat, 2.5 grams saturated fat, no trans fat, 70 milligrams cholesterol, 23 grams carbohydrates, 6 grams dietary fiber, 410 milligrams sodium

Zesty Lemon Chicken

The aromatic oils in citrus zest add so much flavor to foods, and this chicken dish is no exception. Serve this tangy and lean entrée with brown rice pilaf and mixed veggies.

4 six-ounce chicken breasts, skin and fat removed
½ cup fresh lemon juice
2 tablespoons white wine vinegar
½ cup sliced fresh lemon peel
3 teaspoons chopped fresh oregano (or 1 teaspoon crushed dried oregano)
1 medium onion, sliced
¼ teaspoon sea salt
Freshly ground black pepper
Paprika

Place chicken in 13″ × 9″ × 2″ glass baking dish. Mix lemon juice, vinegar, lemon peel, oregano, and onion, and pour over chicken. Cover and marinate in refrigerator for 4 hours or overnight, turning occasionally. When ready to serve, sprinkle with sea salt and add pepper and paprika to taste. Cover baking dish with foil and bake at 325°F for 30 minutes. Uncover and bake for an additional 20 minutes or until chicken is cooked through.

Serves 4 (serving size: 1 chicken breast with sauce)

Servings of fruits and vegetables: ½ vegetable; **cholesterol-lowering phytonutrients:** lutein, sulfides, carotenoids

Nutrition information: 210 calories, 35 grams protein, 4 grams total fat, 1 gram saturated fat, no trans fat, 95 milligrams cholesterol, 9 grams carbohydrates, 2 grams dietary fiber, 200 milligrams sodium

Old-Fashioned Chicken Stew

Comfort food without the guilt! Try our heart-healthy version of an old-fashioned favorite.

8 chicken pieces (breasts or legs)
2 small cloves garlic, minced
1 small yellow onion, chopped
1½ teaspoons sea salt
½ teaspoon freshly ground black pepper
3 medium tomatoes, chopped
1 teaspoon chopped Italian flat-leaf parsley
¼ cup finely chopped celery
2 medium potatoes, peeled and chopped
2 small carrots, chopped
2 bay leaves

Remove the skin and any extra fat from the chicken. In a large skillet, combine chicken, 1 cup water, garlic, onion, salt, pepper, tomatoes, and parsley. Tightly cover and cook over low heat for 25 minutes. Add celery, potatoes, carrots, and bay leaves, and continue to cook for 15 more minutes or until chicken and vegetables are tender. Remove bay leaves before serving.

Serves 8 (serving size: 1 piece of chicken)

Servings of fruits and vegetables: 1½ vegetables; **cholesterol-lowering phytonutrients:** lutein, sulfides, lycopene

Nutrition information: 190 calories, 27 grams protein, 3 grams total fat, 1 gram saturated fat, no trans fat, 65 milligrams cholesterol, 14 grams carbohydrates, 2 grams dietary fiber, 440 milligrams sodium

Grilled Chicken with Chile-Lime Sauce

Also known as a Mexican green tomato, the tomatillo has flavor hints of lemon, apple, and herbs. This zesty chicken dish is heart-healthy fare with Latin flair.

¼ cup extra-virgin olive oil
Juice of 2 limes, divided
¼ teaspoon dried oregano
½ teaspoon freshly ground black pepper
4 4-ounce skinless, boneless chicken breasts
10 to 12 tomatillos, husks removed and halved
½ medium yellow onion, quartered
2 large cloves garlic, chopped fine
2 serrano or jalapeño peppers
2 tablespoons chopped cilantro
¼ teaspoon sea salt
¼ cup low-fat sour cream

Combine the oil, juice from one lime, oregano, and black pepper in a shallow glass baking dish; stir. Place the chicken breasts in the baking dish and turn to coat each side. Cover the dish and refrigerate overnight. Turn the chicken periodically to marinate chicken on both sides.

Put ¼ cup water, tomatillos, and onion into a saucepan. Bring to a gentle boil and simmer uncovered for 10 minutes or until the tomatillos are tender. In a blender, puree the cooked onion, tomatillos, and any remaining water. Add garlic, peppers, cilantro, salt, and remaining lime juice. Blend until all the ingredients are smooth. Place the sauce in a bowl and refrigerate. Place the chicken breasts on a hot grill until cooked through. Place the chicken on a serving platter. Spoon a tablespoon of low-fat sour cream over each chicken breast and top with some of the sauce. Pour the sauce over the sour cream.

Serves 4 (serving size: 1 chicken breast)

Servings of fruits and vegetables: ⅓ vegetable; **cholesterol-lowering phytonutrients:** lutein, sulfides, carotenoids, terpenes

---

Nutrition information: 340 calories, 32 grams protein, 11 grams total fat, 3 grams saturated fat, no trans fat, 80 milligrams cholesterol, 30 grams carbohydrates, 1 gram dietary fiber, 200 milligrams sodium

---

*Q*uick *Chicken Creole*

This is a fast-fix and heart-healthy spicy chicken dish.

Nonstick cooking spray
1 pound boneless, skinless, chicken breasts, cut into 1-inch strips
1 14-ounce can tomatoes, chopped
1 cup low-sodium chili sauce
1½ cups chopped green bell pepper
½ cup chopped celery
¼ cup chopped onion
2 cloves garlic, minced
1 tablespoon fresh basil (or 1 teaspoon dried)
1 tablespoon fresh Italian flat-leaf parsley (or 1 teaspoon dried)
¼ teaspoon crushed red pepper
¼ teaspoon salt
2 cups hot cooked brown rice or whole-wheat pasta

Spray a deep skillet with nonstick spray coating. Preheat pan over medium-high heat. Cook chicken in hot skillet, stirring, for 3 to 5 minutes or until no longer pink. Reduce heat. Add tomatoes and their juice, chili sauce, green pepper, celery, onion, garlic, basil, parsley, red pepper, and salt. Bring to a boil; reduce heat and simmer, covered, for 10 minutes. Serve over hot cooked rice or whole-wheat pasta.

Serves 4 (serving size: 1½ cups)

Servings of fruits and vegetables: 2 vegetables; **cholesterol-lowering phytonutrients:** lycopene, sulfides

Nutrition information: 230 calories, 26 grams protein, 3 grams total fat, 1 gram saturated fat, no trans fat, 65 milligrams cholesterol, 28 grams carbohydrates, 3 grams dietary fiber, 520 milligrams sodium

Chicken Marsala

Imported from Sicily and made from local grapes, Marsala wine has a rich, smoky flavor that ranges from sweet to dry.

⅛ teaspoon black pepper
¼ teaspoon salt
¼ cup flour
4 4-ounce boneless, skinless chicken breasts
1 tablespoon extra-virgin olive oil
½ cup Marsala wine
Juice of ½ lemon
½ cup chicken broth or vegetable broth
½ cup sliced mushrooms
1 tablespoon chopped fresh Italian flat-leaf parsley

Mix together pepper, salt, and flour. Coat chicken with seasoned flour. In a large, heavy-bottomed skillet, heat oil. Place chicken breasts in skillet and brown on both sides. Remove chicken pieces from skillet and set aside. To the skillet, add wine and stir until the wine is heated. Add lemon juice, broth, and mushrooms. Stir to combine, then reduce heat, and cook for about 10 minutes until the sauce is partially reduced.

Return browned chicken breasts to skillet; spoon sauce over the chicken. Cover and cook for about 5 to 10 minutes or until chicken is cooked through. Garnish with parsley.

Serves 4 (serving size: 1 chicken breast with ⅓ cup sauce)

Servings of fruits and vegetables: none; **cholesterol-lowering phytonutrients:** lignans

---

Nutrition information: 240 calories, 24 grams protein, 7 grams total fat, 1 gram saturated fat, no trans fat, 65 milligrams cholesterol, no carbohydrates, 12 grams dietary fiber, 320 milligrams sodium

---

Oven-Fried Chicken

All the taste without the grease!

1 teaspoon poultry seasoning
½ cup skim milk or buttermilk
1½ tablespoons onion powder
1½ tablespoons garlic powder
2 teaspoons black pepper
2 teaspoons crushed dried red pepper flakes
1 teaspoon ground ginger

1 cup crushed cornflakes
8 pieces skinless chicken (4 4-ounce breasts, 4 small
  drumsticks)
Paprika to sprinkle
1 teaspoon vegetable oil (to grease baking pan)

Add ½ teaspoon of poultry seasoning to milk. Combine remaining poultry seasoning, onion powder, garlic powder, black pepper, red pepper flakes, and ground ginger with cornflake crumbs and place in a plastic bag. Wash chicken and pat dry. Dip chicken into milk, shake to remove excess, and then quickly shake in bag with seasoning and crumbs. Refrigerate coated chicken on a cookie sheet for 1 hour. Preheat oven to 350°F.

Remove from refrigerator and sprinkle lightly with paprika for color. Evenly space chicken on greased or parchment-paper-lined baking pan. Cover with aluminum foil and bake 40 minutes. Remove foil and continue baking for an additional 30 to 40 minutes or until the meat can be easily pulled away from the bone with a fork. Crumbs will form a crispy "skin." (Do not turn chicken during baking.)

Serves 8 (serving size: ½ chicken breast or 2 small drumsticks)

Servings of fruits and vegetables: none; **cholesterol-lowering phytonutrients:** sulfides

---

Nutrition information: 180 calories, 25 grams protein, 5 grams total fat, 1.5 grams saturated fat, no trans fat, 70 milligrams cholesterol, 9 grams carbohydrates, 1 gram dietary fiber, 110 milligrams sodium

---

Shanghai Chicken Kabobs

No need to leave home for a tasty trip to another land!

2 pounds boneless, skinless chicken breasts cut into large pieces
Freshly ground black pepper, to taste
8 fresh mushrooms
8 whole white onions, parboiled
2 seedless oranges, quartered
8 canned pineapple chunks, in their own juice
8 cherry tomatoes
1 6-ounce can frozen, concentrated apple juice, thawed
1 cup dry white wine
2 tablespoons low-sodium soy sauce
Dash ground ginger
2 tablespoons vinegar
¼ cup vegetable oil

Cut chicken breasts into 32 pieces. Sprinkle chicken with pepper. Thread eight skewers as follows: chicken, mushroom, chicken, onion, chicken, orange quarter, chicken, pineapple chunk, cherry tomato. Place kabobs in shallow pan. Combine remaining ingredients; spoon over kabobs. Cover and marinate in refrigerator at least 1 hour and up to 6 hours. Drain. Broil 6 inches from heat, 15 minutes on each side, brushing with marinade every 5 minutes. Discard any leftover marinade.

Serves 8 (serving size: 1 chicken breast kabob)

Servings of fruits and vegetables: ⅓ fruit, 1½ vegetables; **cholesterol-lowering phytonutrients:** hesperetin, sulfides, lycopene

---

Nutrition information: 330 calories, 29 grams protein, 10 grams total fat, 2 grams saturated fat, no trans fat, 75 milligrams cholesterol, 24 grams carbohydrates, 2 grams dietary fiber, 210 milligrams sodium

Fish and Seafood

Deep sea protection! As we discussed in Chapter 3, the types of fats we eat play a big role in how our insulin functions. Fish offers heart-healthy and blood-sugar-balancing omega-3 fatty acids for real health!

*T*rout Veracruz

A mild, delicate fish with a sweet flavor and full of heart-helping B vitamins. Enjoy this trout dish often.

> 2 pounds trout fillet, cut into 6 pieces (Any kind of fish can be used.)
> 3 tablespoons fresh lime juice (about 2 limes)
> 1 medium tomato, chopped
> ½ medium yellow onion, chopped
> 3 tablespoons cilantro, chopped
> ½ teaspoon extra-virgin olive oil
> ¼ teaspoon freshly ground black pepper
> ¼ teaspoon salt
> ¼ teaspoon cayenne pepper (optional)

Preheat oven to 350°F. Rinse fish and pat dry. Place in baking dish. In a small bowl, combine lime juice, tomato, onion, cilantro, olive oil, black pepper, salt, and cayenne pepper together and pour over fish. Bake for 15 to 20 minutes or until fork-tender.

Serves 6 (serving size: 1 piece of fish)

Servings of fruits and vegetables: approximately ½ vegetable; **cholesterol-lowering phytonutrients:** sulfides, carotenoids

Nutrition information: 170 calories, 26 grams protein, 6 grams total fat, 1.5 grams saturated fat, no trans fat, 125 milligrams cholesterol, 3 grams carbohydrates, 1 gram dietary fiber, 190 milligrams sodium

Mediterranean Baked Snapper

A firm textured fish with great flavor and very little natural fat, snapper is the perfect complement to these Mediterranean flavors.

2 teaspoons extra-virgin olive oil
1 large yellow onion, sliced
1 16-ounce can whole tomatoes, drained (reserve juice) and chopped
1 bay leaf
1 large clove garlic, minced
1 cup dry white wine
½ cup reserved tomato juice, from canned tomatoes
¼ cup fresh lemon juice
¼ cup fresh orange juice
1 tablespoon freshly grated orange peel
1 teaspoon crushed fennel seeds
½ teaspoon crushed dried oregano
½ teaspoon crushed dried thyme
½ teaspoon crushed dried basil
Freshly ground black pepper, to taste
4 4-ounce snapper fillets (preferable yellowtail)

Heat oil in large nonstick skillet. Add onion, and sauté over medium heat for 5 minutes or until soft. Add tomatoes, bay leaf, garlic, wine, reserved tomato juice, lemon and orange juice, orange peel, fennel seeds, oregano, thyme, basil, and black pepper. Stir well and simmer uncovered for 30 minutes. Preheat oven to 375°F. Arrange fish in 10″ × 6″ baking dish; cover with sauce. Bake, uncovered, about 15 minutes or until fish flakes easily.

Serves 4 (serving size: 1 fillet with sauce)

Servings of fruits and vegetables: approximately 1½ vegetables; **cholesterol-lowering phytonutrients:** lycopene, lignans, sulfides

Nutrition information: 230 calories, 25 grams protein, 4 grams total fat, 0.5 gram saturated fat, no trans fat, 40 milligrams cholesterol, 19 grams carbohydrates, 2 grams dietary fiber, 560 milligrams sodium

Grouper Veronique

Veronique is a term that describes dishes garnished with seedless white grapes. This tasty treat helps to keep your heart healthy and cholesterol under control. Be sure your baking dish can stand the heat—it will be used under the broiler!

Nonstick cooking spray
4 4-ounce grouper fillets
¼ teaspoon sea salt
⅛ teaspoon freshly ground black pepper
¼ cup dry white wine
¼ cup chicken broth or vegetable broth
1 tablespoon fresh lemon juice

1 tablespoon canola-based margarine (nonhydrogenated)
2 tablespoons flour
¾ cup low-fat (1 percent) or skim milk
½ cup seedless white grapes

Preheat oven to 350°F. Spray 10″ × 6″ baking dish with non-stick cooking spray. Place fish in pan and sprinkle with salt and pepper. Mix wine, broth, and lemon juice in small bowl and pour over fish. Cover with foil and bake for 15 minutes. Melt margarine in small saucepan. Remove from heat and blend in flour. Gradually add milk and cook over medium-low heat, stirring constantly until thickened. Remove fish from oven and carefully pour liquid from baking dish into cream sauce, stirring until blended. Pour sauce over fish and sprinkle with grapes. Broil about 4 inches from heat for 5 minutes or until sauce starts to brown.

Serves 4 (serving size: 1 fillet with ⅓ cup sauce)

Servings of fruits and vegetables: none; **cholesterol-lowering phytonutrients:** none

Nutrition information: 190 calories, 24 grams protein, 5 grams total fat, 0.5 gram saturated fat, no trans fat, 40 milligrams cholesterol, 11 grams carbohydrates, no dietary fiber, 360 milligrams sodium

Oven-Fried Catfish

Catfish is a firm textured fish that's low in fat and mild in flavor. It doesn't have to be deep fried to be enjoyed. Try this heart-healthy recipe and you'll agree. Serve with collard greens and black-eyed peas.

2 pounds catfish fillets, cut into 6 pieces
1 tablespoon fresh lemon juice
¼ cup skim milk or 1 percent buttermilk
2 drops hot pepper sauce
1 teaspoon minced fresh garlic
¼ teaspoon ground white pepper
¼ teaspoon sea salt
¼ teaspoon onion powder
½ cup crushed cornflakes
1 tablespoon vegetable oil (for greasing baking dish)
1 lemon, cut in wedges

Preheat oven to 475°F. Brush fillets with lemon juice and pat dry. Combine milk, hot pepper sauce, and garlic; set aside. Combine pepper, salt, and onion powder with cornflake crumbs and place on a plate. Let fillets sit in milk briefly. Remove and coat fillets on both sides with seasoned crumbs. Let stand for 30 minutes until coating sticks to each side of fish. Arrange on lightly oiled shallow baking dish. Bake for 20 minutes on middle rack without turning. To serve, cut into 6 pieces and serve with fresh lemon.

Serves 6 (serving size: 1 piece of fish)

Servings of fruits and vegetables: none; **cholesterol-lowering phytonutrients:** none

Nutrition information: 180 calories, 27 grams protein, 6 grams total fat, 1 gram saturated fat, no trans fat, 70 milligrams cholesterol, 4 grams carbohydrates, no dietary fiber, 250 milligrams sodium

Scallop Kabobs

High in protein, low in fat, these scallops make for a sweet, tasty grill alternative when only the best will do!

3 medium green bell peppers, cut into 1½-inch squares
1½ pounds fresh sea scallops
1 pint cherry tomatoes
¼ cup dry white wine
¼ cup vegetable oil
3 tablespoons fresh lemon juice
Dash garlic powder
Black pepper to taste

Heat grill or broiler. Parboil green peppers for 2 minutes. Thread peppers, scallops, and cherry tomatoes on four skewers, alternating pepper, scallop, tomato. In a small bowl combine wine, oil, lemon juice, garlic powder, and black pepper, mixing well. Brush kabobs with mixture and place on grill (or under broiler). Grill or broil for 15 minutes, turning and basting frequently.

Serves 4 (serving size: 1 scallop kabob)

Servings of fruits and vegetables: 2 vegetables; **cholesterol-lowering phytonutrients:** lutein, lycopene

Nutrition information: 310 calories, 30 grams protein, 15 grams total fat, 2 grams saturated fat, no trans fat, 55 milligrams cholesterol, 14 grams carbohydrates, 2 grams dietary fiber, 370 milligrams sodium

Sole Florentine

Nicknamed Jupiter's sandal because of the elongated oval shape of this flatfish, sole has been popular since the Romans.

Nonstick cooking spray
1 teaspoon extra-virgin olive oil
½ pound fresh mushrooms, sliced
½ pound fresh spinach, cleaned, stemmed, and chopped
¼ teaspoon crushed dried oregano leaves
1 large clove garlic, minced
4 6-ounce sole fillets or other white fish
2 tablespoons sherry
4 ounces part-skim mozzarella cheese, grated

Preheat oven to 400°F. Spray a 10″ × 6″ baking dish with nonstick cooking spray. Heat oil in skillet; sauté mushrooms until tender, for about 3 minutes. Add spinach and continue cooking for about 1 minute or until spinach is just barely wilted. Remove from heat; drain liquid into prepared baking dish. Add oregano and garlic to drained sautéed vegetables; stir to mix ingredients. Divide vegetable mixture evenly among fillets, placing filling in center of each fillet. Roll fillet around mixture and place seam side down in prepared baking dish. Sprinkle with sherry, then mozzarella cheese. Bake for 15 to 20 minutes or until fish flakes easily. Lift out with a slotted spoon.

Serves 4 (serving size: 1 fillet roll)

Servings of fruits and vegetables: 3 vegetables; **cholesterol-lowering phytonutrients:** lutein, lycopene

Nutrition information: 280 calories, 42 grams protein, 10 grams total fat, 4 grams saturated fat, no trans fat, 95 milligrams cholesterol, 6 grams carbohydrates, 2 grams dietary fiber, 420 milligrams sodium

βroiled Mahimahi with Red Bell Pepper Sauce

A Florida favorite, mahimahi is a light fish that supplies a boatload of heart-helping B vitamins. Red bell peppers add a sweet flavor and fresh color and a perfect sauce complement to this fish dish.

⅙ cup extra-virgin olive oil
⅓ cup unsalted pumpkin seeds, toasted
¾ cup chopped fresh basil
2 cloves garlic, crushed
1 large red bell pepper, diced
2 4-ounce mahimahi fillets

In a medium saucepan, heat oil over medium low. Crush pumpkin seeds using a mortar and pestle. Heat a small saucepan of water to boiling and add basil to blanch. (This helps to retain the green color.) Quickly remove the blanched basil, drain, and set aside. Add crushed pumpkin seeds, garlic, bell pepper, and basil to oil over medium-low heat and cook for 10 minutes. Brush mahimahi fillets with a small amount of pepper sauce. Place under broiler for 5 to 8 minutes until juices run clear and fish is white throughout. Top mahimahi with remaining bell pepper sauce and serve.

Serves 2 (serving size: 1 fillet)

Servings of fruits and vegetables: 1 vegetable; **cholesterol-lowering phytonutrients:** terpenes, lycopene, allicin, sulfides

Nutrition information: 490 calories, 35 grams protein, 36 grams total fat, 6 grams saturated fat, no trans fat, 83 milligrams cholesterol, 12 grams carbohydrates, 4 grams dietary fiber, 109 milligrams sodium

Dijon Cod

Dijon mustard adds a spicy pungency to this fish dish that is quick to prepare and beneficial to the heart.

Nonstick cooking spray
1 small yellow onion, diced
4 plum tomatoes, diced
⅓ cup white wine
4 4-ounce cod fillets
Pinch sea salt
¾ cup whole-grain bread crumbs
2 tablespoons chopped fresh Italian flat-leaf parsley
1 tablespoon canola margarine
2 teaspoons spicy Dijon mustard

Preheat oven to 400°F. Coat a large oven-safe skillet with nonstick spray and add the onion and tomatoes, heating over medium. Roast on the stove top for 10 minutes, stirring occasionally. Increase heat to medium high, and add the wine. Arrange cod in a single layer over mixture. Sprinkle with salt. In a small bowl, combine bread crumbs, parsley, canola margarine, and mustard. Sprinkle over fillets, pressing firmly into fish. Bake for 15 to 20 minutes or until fish flakes easily.

Serves 4 (serving size: 1 fillet)

Servings of fruits and vegetables: 1 vegetable; **cholesterol-lowering phytonutrients:** lycopene

Nutrition information: 190 calories, 21 grams protein, 5 grams total fat, 0.5 gram saturated fat, no trans fat, 45 milligrams cholesterol, 16 grams carbohydrates, 2 grams dietary fiber, 330 milligrams sodium

*P*esto Salmon

Tired of simply grilling or baking salmon? Pesto is an uncooked sauce made primarily from fresh basil and nuts with oil. This version uses almonds and a lot less oil—for a flavorful but healthier version.

3 tablespoons vegetable broth
1½ cups fresh basil leaves
1 tablespoon slivered almonds
1 tablespoon fresh lemon juice
2 teaspoons grated Parmesan cheese
2 teaspoons extra-virgin olive oil
Pinch sea salt
Freshly ground black pepper, to taste
1 large clove garlic
4 4-ounce salmon steaks or fillets
Basil sprigs and lemon wedges for garnish

Make the pesto by placing the broth, basil, almonds, lemon juice, Parmesan, olive oil, salt, pepper, and garlic in a food processor, pulsing until pureed. Place the salmon on a plate. Spoon approximately 3 tablespoons of the pesto over the salmon, and turn to coat. Cover with plastic wrap, and let stand for 15 minutes at room temperature. Place the salmon in an oiled broiler pan. Broil the salmon approximately 4 to 5 inches from broiler element for 6 to 8 minutes, or until opaque in the center. Transfer to plates; garnish with fresh basil and lemon wedges.

Serves 4 (serving size: 1 fillet with sauce)

Servings of fruits and vegetables: none; **cholesterol-lowering phytonutrients:** terpenes

Nutrition information: 250 calories, 24 grams protein, 16 grams total fat, 3 grams saturated fat, no trans fat, 65 milligrams cholesterol, 2 grams carbohydrates, 1 gram dietary fiber, 230 milligrams sodium

Sesame and Black Pepper–Encrusted Tuna

Sesame seeds also come in shades of red, brown, or black, but you'll want to use the more traditional ivory colored ones for this encrusting.

    2 4-ounce fresh tuna steaks
    2 tablespoons toasted (Oriental) sesame oil
    1 medium gingerroot, peeled and grated
    4 blades of lemongrass, chopped fine
    4 tablespoons sesame seeds

¼ cup black peppercorns, crushed
Steamed brown rice
Steamed mixed Asian vegetables

Coat tuna steaks with oil. Rub with ginger and lemongrass. Press half of the sesame seeds and half of the peppercorns onto each side of the tuna, pressing to encrust. Flip and coat other side of tuna with remaining sesame seeds and peppercorns. Heat grill to high, and cook for 4 to 6 minutes per side. Serve with brown rice and mixed Asian vegetables.

Serves 2 (serving size: 1 fillet)

Servings of fruits and vegetables: none; **cholesterol-lowering phytonutrients:** sesamin

Nutrition information: 300 calories, 13 grams protein, 24 grams total fat, 2.5 grams saturated fat, no trans fat, 15 milligrams cholesterol, 7 grams carbohydrates, 3 grams dietary fiber, 460 milligrams sodium

Garden Entrées

On the lighter side, these meals are a perfect example of how to give your vegetables center stage without sacrificing flavor.

N'Orleans Red Beans and Rice

Red beans and rice is a tradition down in New Orleans, but there's no reason why you can't enjoy it anytime in your hometown. This Southern-style meal is packed with phytoestrogens and quercetin, and you'll learn to love your legumes!

1 pound dry red beans
1½ cups chopped yellow onion
1 cup chopped celery
4 bay leaves
1 cup chopped green bell pepper
3 tablespoons chopped fresh garlic
3 tablespoons chopped Italian flat-leaf parsley
2 teaspoons crushed dried thyme
1 teaspoon sea salt
1 teaspoon freshly ground black pepper
4 cups hot cooked brown rice

Pick through beans to remove any stones or shriveled beans; rinse thoroughly. In a large pot combine beans, 2 quarts water, onion, celery, and bay leaves. Bring to a boil; reduce heat. Cover and cook over low heat for about 1½ hours or until beans are tender. Stir. Mash beans against side of pan. Add green pepper, garlic, parsley, thyme, salt, and black pepper. Cook, uncovered, over low heat until creamy, about 30 minutes. Remove bay leaves. Serve with hot cooked brown rice.

Serves 8 (serving size: 1¼ cups)

Servings of fruits and vegetables: 1 vegetable; **cholesterol-lowering phytonutrients:** phytoestrogens, quercetin, allicin, sulfides

---

Nutrition information: 220 calories, 15 grams protein, no total fat, no saturated fat, no trans fat, no cholesterol, 40 grams carbohydrates, 15 grams dietary fiber, 270 milligrams sodium

---

Garden Fresh Pasta Sauce

For a heart-healthy Italian meal, enjoy this dish fresh from your garden or from the produce department of your favorite market!

    2 tablespoons extra-virgin olive oil
    2 small yellow onions, chopped
    3 large cloves garlic, chopped
    1¼ cups sliced zucchini
    1 tablespoon dried oregano
    1 tablespoon dried basil
    1 8-ounce can tomato sauce
    1 6-ounce can tomato paste
    2 medium tomatoes, chopped
    12 ounces whole-wheat spaghetti, cooked (or other whole-
        grain pasta), to serve

In a medium skillet, heat oil. Sauté onions, garlic, and zucchini in oil for 5 minutes over medium heat. Add remaining ingredients and 1 cup of water and simmer, covered, for 45 minutes. Serve over spaghetti.

Serves 6 (serving size: ¾ cup of sauce with ½ cup spaghetti)

Servings of fruits and vegetables: 2 vegetables; **cholesterol-lowering phytonutrients:** lycopene, allicin, sulfides

---

Nutrition information: 110 calories, 3 grams protein, 5 grams total fat, 0.5 gram saturated fat, no trans fat, 95 milligrams cholesterol, 15 grams carbohydrates, 3 grams dietary fiber, 430 milligrams sodium

---

Zucchini Lasagna

This heart-healthy meal full of lycopene and allicin proves that you can still have your lasagna and eat it, too. If you always add salt to the water when you're boiling pasta, get in the habit of avoiding it. You won't miss the added salt, it serves no benefit to the boiling process, and you'll cut back on the added sodium in the process.

> Vegetable oil spray
> ¾ cup grated part-skim mozzarella cheese
> ¼ cup grated Parmesan cheese
> 1½ cups fat-free cottage cheese
> 2½ cups no-salt-added tomato sauce
> 2 teaspoons dried basil
> 2 teaspoons dried oregano
> ¼ cup chopped yellow onion
> 1 large clove garlic
> ⅛ teaspoon freshly ground black pepper
> ½ pound cooked lasagna noodles (in unsalted water)
> 1½ cups sliced zucchini

Preheat oven to 350°F. Lightly spray a 9″ × 13″ baking dish with vegetable oil spray. In a small bowl, combine ⅛ cup mozzarella and 1 tablespoon Parmesan cheese. Set aside. In a medium bowl, combine remaining mozzarella and Parmesan cheese with all of the cottage cheese. Mix well and set aside.

Combine tomato sauce with basil, oregano, onion, garlic, and pepper. Spread a thin layer of tomato sauce in the bottom of the baking dish. Add a third of the noodles in a single layer. Spread half of the cottage cheese mixture on top. Add a layer of zucchini. Repeat layering. Add a thin coating of sauce. Top with noodles, sauce, and reserved cheese mixture. Cover with aluminum foil. Bake for 30 to 40 minutes. Cool for 10 to 15 minutes. Cut into six portions.

Serves 6 (serving size: ⅙ of recipe)

Servings of fruits and vegetables: 3 vegetables; **cholesterol-lowering phytonutrients:** lycopene, terpenes, sulfides, allicin

Nutrition information: 276 calories, 5 grams protein, 5 grams total fat, 2 grams saturated fat, 11 milligrams cholesterol, 5 grams carbohydrates, no dietary fiber, 380 milligrams sodium

---

Caribbean Black Beans and Rice

Another great version of beans and rice, this time from the tropics.

1 pound dry black beans
1 medium green bell pepper, chopped coarse
1½ cups chopped yellow onion
1 tablespoon canola oil
2 bay leaves

1 large clove garlic, minced
½ teaspoon sea salt
1 tablespoon apple cider vinegar (or lemon juice)
6 cups brown rice, cooked in unsalted water
1 lemon, cut into wedges

Pick through beans and remove any stones or shriveled beans. Soak beans overnight in 7 cups of cold water. Drain and rinse. In large soup pot or Dutch oven stir together beans, water, green pepper, onion, oil, bay leaves, garlic, and salt. Cover and boil 1 hour. Reduce heat and simmer, covered, for 1½ hours or until beans are very tender. Stir occasionally and add additional water as needed. Remove about ⅓ of the beans, mash, and return to pot. Stir and heat through. Remove bay leaves and stir in vinegar or lemon juice when ready to serve. Serve over rice. Garnish with lemon wedges.

Serves 6 (serving size: 1 cup)

Servings of fruits and vegetables: none; **cholesterol-lowering phytonutrients:** lycopene, phytoestrogens, quercetin, sulfides

---

Nutrition information: 190 calories, 8 grams protein, 2 grams total fat, no saturated fat, no trans fat, no cholesterol, 36 grams carbohydrates, 7 grams dietary fiber, 55 milligrams sodium

---

Summer Vegetable Stew

If you only think of stew in the winter, think again. What better time to take advantage of the health benefits and fresh flavors of summer vegetables.

1 cup low-sodium vegetable broth
2 cups sliced white potatoes
2 cups sliced carrots
4 cups chunked zucchini
1 cup chunked summer squash
1 15-ounce can sweet corn, rinsed and drained (or 2 ears
 fresh corn, 1½ cups)
1 teaspoon dried thyme
2 large cloves garlic, minced
1 scallion, chopped
½ small hot pepper (such as jalapeño), chopped
1 cup coarsely chopped yellow onion
1 cup broccoli florets
1 cup seeded and diced tomatoes

Heat 3 cups water and vegetable broth in a large pot and bring to a boil. Add potatoes and carrots to the broth, and simmer for 5 minutes. Add the remaining ingredients except for the tomatoes, and continue cooking for 15 minutes over medium heat. Remove four chunks of squash and puree in blender. Return pureed mixture to pot, and let cook for 10 more minutes. Add tomatoes, and cook for another 5 minutes. Remove from heat and let sit for 15 minutes to allow stew to thicken.

Serves 8 (serving size: 1¼ cups)

Servings of fruits and vegetables: 3 vegetables; **cholesterol-lowering phytonutrients:** lycopene, allicin, quercetin, carotenoids

Nutrition information: 120 calories, 4 grams protein, 0.5 gram total fat, no saturated fat, no trans fat, no cholesterol, 28 grams carbohydrates, 4 grams dietary fiber, 250 milligrams sodium

Roasted Italian Vegetable Terrine

Interchangeable with the term pâté, this traditionally packed ground cooked meat preparation is delicious with roasted vegetables instead. Roasting the vegetables gives them a hearty flavor that complements the herbs while providing nutrients and fiber to help you cut cholesterol.

1 28-ounce can whole tomatoes
1 medium yellow onion, sliced
½ pound fresh green beans, sliced
½ pound fresh okra, cut into ½-inch pieces (or ½ of a
    10-ounce package frozen okra)
¾ cup finely chopped green bell pepper
2 tablespoons fresh lemon juice
1 teaspoon chopped fresh basil (or 1 teaspoon dried basil,
    crushed)
1½ teaspoons chopped fresh oregano leaves (or ½ teaspoon
    dried oregano, crushed)
3 medium (7-inch-long) zucchini, cut into 1-inch cubes
1 medium eggplant, peeled and cut into 1-inch cubes
2 tablespoons grated Parmesan cheese

Preheat oven to 325°F. Drain and coarsely chop tomatoes, reserving liquid. Mix together tomatoes and reserved liquid, onion, green beans, okra, green pepper, lemon juice, and herbs. Cover and bake for 15 minutes. Mix in zucchini and eggplant and continue baking, covered, 60 to 70 more minutes or until vegetables are tender. Stir occasionally. Sprinkle top with Parmesan cheese just before serving.

Serves 18 (serving size: ½ cup)

Servings of fruits and vegetables: 2 vegetables; **cholesterol-lowering phytonutrients:** lycopene, quercetin

Nutrition information: 30 calories, 2 grams protein, no total fat, no trans fat, no saturated fat, no cholesterol, 6 grams carbohydrates, 3 grams dietary fiber, 65 milligrams sodium

Roasted Red Pepper and Pesto Sandwich

This quick sandwich is loaded with lycopene to fend off heart-harming free radicals. Roasting red peppers gives them a sweet and more flavorful taste.

1 tablespoon soy mayonnaise
2 teaspoons basil pesto
1 slice whole-grain bread, cut in half horizontally
2 tablespoons sun-dried tomato pesto
¼ cup roasted red peppers
½ cup crumbled feta cheese
½ cup fresh basil leaves

In a small bowl, mix together mayonnaise and basil pesto; spread onto one half of bread. Spread other half with sun-dried tomato pesto. Arrange roasted red peppers on bottom piece. Cover with feta cheese, then fresh basil. Top with remaining slice of bread.

Serves 1 (serving size: 1 sandwich)

Servings of fruits and vegetables: ¹/₂ vegetable; **cholesterol-lowering phytonutrients:** lycopene

Nutrition information: 490 calories, 19 grams protein, 29 grams total fat, 9 grams saturated fat, no trans fat, 30 milligrams cholesterol, 37 grams carbohydrates, 6 grams dietary fiber, 1,260 milligrams sodium

*β*lack Bean Burritos

Who says Mexican food can't be healthy? All the flavor with a lot less fat, this black bean burrito will become part of your south-of-the-border celebrations, even if that just means a weeknight dinner!

> 2 16-ounce cans black beans, drained and rinsed
> 1 tablespoon chopped canned chipotle chilies with some of the adobo sauce
> 1½ teaspoons ground cumin
> 1½ cups sliced scallions
> ⅓ cup chopped cilantro leaves
> 6 10-inch flour tortillas, warmed
> ½ cup shredded low-fat Monterey Jack cheese
> 3 cups shredded lettuce
> Prepared salsa and guacamole (optional)
> 4 cilantro sprigs (optional)

In a large saucepan, heat the beans, chipotles, and cumin over medium heat, stirring occasionally, until simmering. Stir in the scallions and chopped cilantro; continue to simmer 2 minutes. To assemble, spoon about ½ cup bean mixture on center of each tortilla. Top with equal amounts of the cheese and lettuce. Fold bottom edge up over filling. Fold right and left sides to center, overlapping edges. Serve with the salsa and guacamole, and garnish with the cilantro sprigs, if desired.

Serves 6 (serving size: 1 burrito)

Servings of fruits and vegetables: ½ vegetable; **cholesterol-lowering phytonutrients:** phytoestrogens, sulfides

Nutrition information: 380 calories, 17 grams protein, 7 grams total fat, 2.5 grams saturated fat, no trans fat, 5 milligrams cholesterol, 55 grams carbohydrates, 16 grams dietary fiber, 970 milligrams sodium

Fajita Burgers

This cholesterol-crushing veggie burger has a Latin accent.

1 teaspoon vegetable oil, divided
½ medium green or red bell pepper, cut into strips
1 small yellow onion, sliced thin
¼ teaspoon chili powder
2 frozen meatless cheeseburgers
2 8-inch flour tortillas, warmed

Heat ½ teaspoon of the oil in large nonstick skillet on medium heat. Add pepper, onion, and chili powder; cook and stir 5 minutes or until tender-crisp. Remove from pan. Add remaining ½ teaspoon oil to skillet. Add cheeseburgers; cook 4 minutes. Turn burgers; top with vegetables. Cook an additional 4 minutes; cut burgers in half. Place two burger halves on each tortilla; top with vegetables.

Serves 2 (serving size: 1 burger)

Servings of fruits and vegetables: 1 vegetable; **cholesterol-lowering phytonutrients:** lycopene

Nutrition information: 280 calories, 19 grams protein, 11 grams total fat, 3 grams saturated fat, no trans fat, 10 milligrams cholesterol, 27 grams carbohydrates, 7 grams dietary fiber, 460 milligrams sodium

Portobello Pizza

Crustless wonders, these pizzas are sure to please the palate and promote a healthy heart. The reduced moisture of this large, flavorful mushroom creates a dense, meaty texture.

> 1 teaspoon extra-virgin olive oil
> 1 large clove garlic, minced
> 4 portobello mushroom caps, cleaned
> Vegetable oil spray
> Pinch salt
> Pinch freshly ground black pepper
> 12 ounces low-fat mozzarella cheese, sliced or shredded
> 10 fresh basil leaves
> 2 medium fresh tomatoes, sliced and roasted or grilled
> Oregano leaves (optional)

Preheat oven to 450°F. Combine the oil and garlic in a small bowl, and rub the mushroom caps on all sides with the mixture. Place the caps, top side down, in a circle on an oiled baking sheet. Season with the salt and pepper. Arrange the cheese, basil, and tomato slices alternately in a circle on top of the mushrooms.

Sprinkle with the oregano, if desired. Bake until the cheese melts, about 3 minutes.

Serves 4 (serving size: 1 mushroom with topping)

Servings of fruits and vegetables: 3 vegetables; **cholesterol-lowering phytonutrients:** lycopene, allicin, lignans

Nutrition information: 160 calories, 15 grams protein, 6 grams total fat, 3 grams saturated fat, no trans fat, 15 milligrams cholesterol, 10 grams carbohydrates, 2 grams dietary fiber, 320 milligrams sodium

Drinks and Desserts

Who says dessert can't be healthy? Try our smoothies, muffins, and other desserts to please your palate without guilt.

Tropical Fruit Compote

Enjoy a taste of the tropics any time of day with this perfect combination of fruit flavors.

¼ cup pineapple juice
2 teaspoons fresh lemon juice
1 piece lemon peel
½ teaspoon vanilla extract
1 pineapple, cored and peeled, cut into 8 slices
2 mangoes, peeled, pitted, and each cut into 8 pieces
3 bananas, peeled and each cut into 8 diagonal pieces
Fresh mint leaves

In a saucepan combine ¾ cup water with the pineapple juice, lemon juice, lemon peel, and vanilla extract. Bring to a boil, then reduce the heat and add the fruit. Cook at a very low heat for 5 minutes. Pour the syrup in a cup. Remove the lemon rind, and cool the cooked fruit for 2 hours. To serve the compote, arrange the fruit in serving dishes and pour a few teaspoons of syrup over the fruit. Garnish with mint leaves. Serve with low-fat yogurt.

Serves 8 (serving size: 1 cup)

Servings of fruits and vegetables: 2 fruits; **cholesterol-lowering phytonutrients:** carotenoids, limonene

Nutrition information: 110 calories, 1 gram protein, no total fat, no saturated fat, no cholesterol, 27 grams carbohydrates, 3 grams dietary fiber, no sodium

Peach and Berry Tart

Anthocyanin-rich berries meet up with cholesterol-cutting carotenoids for a dish that's easy on the heart and taste buds. The oats and whole-wheat flour add a nutty crunch to this fresh fruit tart.

Vegetable oil spray
⅔ cup rolled oats
1 teaspoon ground cinnamon
½ cup whole-wheat flour
1 tablespoon light brown sugar
¼ teaspoon baking soda
2 tablespoons canola oil
2 tablespoons plain, nonfat yogurt, plus more as needed
1 pint berries (strawberries, blackberries, raspberries), sliced
1 pound fresh peaches, sliced (or 1½ cups sliced frozen peaches)
¼ cup all-fruit spread
½ teaspoon vanilla extract (or 1 whole vanilla bean)

Preheat oven to 375°F; lightly coat a cookie sheet with oil or line with parchment paper. Combine oats, cinnamon, flour, brown sugar, and baking soda in a bowl, mixing well with a fork. Stir in oil and yogurt, adding more yogurt if dough is too stiff.

Pat dough evenly onto cookie sheet in a 10-inch circle, and use a 9-inch pan to make the circle perfect, trimming around the outside with a knife. Pinch the rim to ¼ inch high; bake 15 minutes or until crust is firm and golden. Set aside to cool; transfer to a serving plate.

Meanwhile, combine berries, peaches, fruit spread, and vanilla in a microwave-safe bowl; microwave 10 seconds to melt the spread. Spoon the fruit mixture onto the crust; refrigerate 30 minutes. Slice into eight wedges, and serve.

Serves 8 (serving size: 1 slice)

Servings of fruits and vegetables: 1½ fruits; **cholesterol-lowering phytonutrients:** carotenoids, anthocyanins

---

Nutrition information: 160 calories, 3 grams protein, 4.5 grams total fat, no saturated fat, no trans fat, no cholesterol, 29 grams carbohydrates, 5 grams dietary fiber, no sodium

---

Carotene Cooler

What a power-packed refresher! Shop for the ripest mangoes (or ripen them in a paper bag for a few days on your kitchen counter). Cholesterol-cutting carotenoids take center stage in this light and frothy smoothie.

> 1 cup chopped fresh mango
> 1 cup ice
> 1 cup low-fat yogurt
> 2 cups orange juice
> 2 teaspoons flaxseed oil

Put all ingredients into a blender. Blend until foamy. Serve immediately.

Serves 2 (serving size: ¾ cup)

Servings of fruits and vegetables: 2⅓ fruits; **cholesterol-lowering phytonutrients:** carotenoids

Nutrition information: 250 calories, 10 grams protein, 7 grams total fat, 1.5 grams saturated fat, no trans fat, 10 milligrams cholesterol, 39 grams carbohydrates, 2 grams dietary fiber, 110 milligrams sodium

*A*pple and Cranberry Crisp

Fiber-full apples and anthocyanin-rich cranberries nestle into this comforting crisp.

½ cup turbinado or date sugar
3 tablespoons plus ¼ cup whole-wheat flour
1 teaspoon grated lemon peel
¾ teaspoon fresh lemon juice
5 cups sliced unpeeled apples
1 cup cranberries
⅔ cup old-fashioned rolled oats
⅓ cup light or dark brown sugar, packed
2 teaspoons ground cinnamon
1 tablespoon canola margarine, melted

Preheat oven to 375°F. To prepare filling, in a medium bowl combine sugar, 3 tablespoons of the flour, and lemon peel; mix well. Add lemon juice, apples, and cranberries; stir to mix. Spoon into a 6-cup baking dish. To prepare topping, in a small bowl, combine oats, brown sugar, remaining ¼ cup flour, and cinnamon. Add melted margarine; stir to mix. Sprinkle topping over filling. Bake for approximately 40 to 50 minutes or until filling is bubbly and top is brown. Serve warm or at room temperature.

Serves 6 (serving size: 1¾-by-2-inch piece)

Servings of fruits and vegetables: 1 fruit; **cholesterol-lowering phytonutrients:** carotenoids, anthocyanins

Nutrition information: 260 calories, 3 grams protein, 3.5 grams total fat, no saturated fat, no trans fat, no cholesterol, 58 grams carbohydrates, 6 grams dietary fiber, 5 milligrams sodium

Berry Blast

An antioxidant-rich delight, this will be perfect with your whole-grain cereal for breakfast or as a post-workout refresher. Frozen unsweetened berries work well when fresh are not in season.

    2 cups mixed berries (raspberries, blueberries, strawberries)
    1 cup low-fat yogurt
    1 cup cranberry juice

Put all ingredients in a blender. Whirl until smooth. Serve.
Note: for a thicker drink plus omega-3 fatty acids and protein, add 1 tablespoon flaxseed meal or hempseed meal.

Serves 2 (serving size: 1 cup)

Servings of fruits and vegetables: 4 fruits; **cholesterol-lowering phytonutrients:** anthocyanins

Nutrition information: 240 calories, 10 grams protein, 2 grams total fat, 1 gram saturated fat, no trans fat, 10 milligrams cholesterol, 54 grams carbohydrates, 8 grams dietary fiber, 105 milligrams sodium

Cinnamon Raisin Scones

This is a heart-healthy alternative to the coffeehouse variety. The secret to tender scones? Handle the dough lightly.

Vegetable oil spray
¼ teaspoon sea salt
½ cup apple juice or vanilla soy milk
½ cup honey
½ cup seedless raisins
½ teaspoon baking soda
1½ cups oat flour (or 1 cup old-fashioned rolled oats buzzed in a food processor)
1½ cups whole-wheat pastry flour
1 tablespoon baking powder
1 teaspoon cinnamon
⅓ cup canola oil

Preheat oven to 350°F. Oil cookie sheet. Mix all remaining ingredients in a large mixing bowl. Drop tablespoon-size spoonfuls of batter onto cookie sheet, leaving 1 inch between each. Bake 15 minutes.

Serves 12 (serving size: 1 scone)

Servings of fruits and vegetables: ⅓ fruit; **cholesterol-lowering phytonutrients:** phytoestrogens, beta-glucan

Nutrition information: 230 calories, 3 grams protein, 8 grams total fat, 0.5 gram saturated fat, no trans fat, 95 milligrams cholesterol, 39 grams carbohydrates, 3 grams dietary fiber, 170 milligrams sodium

Flavonoid Freeze

Berries and grapes team up to clear the arteries and bury cholesterol. Use either lite or regular silken tofu for this recipe.

    1 cup purple grape juice or red wine
    1 cup mixed berries (raspberries, strawberries, blueberries,
        pitted dark cherries)
    ½ cup silken tofu

Place all ingredients in a blender. Puree until smooth. Serve.

Serves 2 (serving size: 1 cup)

Servings of fruits and vegetables: approximately 1½ fruits; **cholesterol-lowering phytonutrients:** phytoestrogens, anthocyanins, resveratrol

Nutrition information: 150 calories, 6 grams protein, 3 grams total fat, no saturated fat, no trans fat, no cholesterol, 29 grams carbohydrates, 2 grams dietary fiber, 10 milligrams sodium

Zesty Green Tea Cooler

Turn on the kettle and turn up the tannins in your diet to lower cholesterol and protect your heart. Green tea is produced from leaves that are steamed and dried but not fermented, making it closer to the taste of a fresh tea leaf.

6 green tea bags
Juice of 1 lemon
3 teaspoons lemon zest
2 teaspoons crushed dried mint leaves
Fresh mint leaves and lemon wedges for garnish

Place 6 cups water in coffeepot. Open tea bags and pour contents into coffee filter along with lemon zest and mint leaves. Brew. Pour Zesty Green Tea into a pitcher, add lemon juice, and refrigerate until chilled. Serve with fresh mint leaves and a lemon wedge.

Serves 6 (serving size: 1 cup)

Servings of fruits and vegetables: none; **cholesterol-lowering phytonutrients:** tannins

Nutrition information: 5 calories, no protein, no total fat, no saturated fat, no cholesterol, 1 gram carbohydrates, no dietary fiber, no sodium

Spicy Cinnamon Chai

This spicy, warming, antioxidant drink benefits the heart and is delicious any time of day.

6 chai tea bags
2 cinnamon sticks, crushed (or 1 teaspoon ground cinnamon)
1 teaspoon cardamom seeds
6 cups spring water
Honey, to taste

Open tea bags and place contents in a coffee filter with cinnamon and cardamom. Place coffee filter in coffeepot. Add water to coffeepot reservoir. Brew tea and serve with honey.

Serves 6 (serving size: 1 cup)

Servings of fruits and vegetables: none; **cholesterol-lowering phytonutrients:** none

Nutrition information: 5 calories, no protein, no total fat, no saturated fat, no cholesterol, 3 grams carbohydrates, no dietary fiber, no sodium

Chocolate Smoothie

Have your chocolate and drink it, too! The berries, mint, and cocoa in this smoothie provide heart-healthy antioxidant phytonutrients and heavenly taste. Grab a straw and try it for dessert tonight.

¾ cup chocolate soy milk
1¼ cups frozen, unsweetened raspberries
½ medium banana, sliced
¾ cup chocolate sorbet
2 tablespoons fresh mint, chopped

Combine the soy milk, raspberries, and banana in a blender. Add the sorbet and mint. Blend until smooth.

Serves 2 (serving size: approximately ½ cup)

Servings of fruits and vegetables: 1 fruit; **cholesterol-lowering phytonutrients:** phytoestrogens

Nutrition information: 200 calories, 5 grams protein, 2.5 grams total fat, no saturated fat, no trans fat, no cholesterol, 43 grams carbohydrates, 9 grams dietary fiber, 65 milligrams sodium

Appendix
Converting to Metrics

Measurement Conversions

We have included the following tables so you can easily convert measuring ingredients.

Volume Measurement Conversions	
U.S.	**Metric**
¼ teaspoon	1.25 ml
½ teaspoon	2.5 ml
¾ teaspoon	3.75 ml
1 teaspoon	5 ml
1 tablespoon	15 ml
¼ cup	62.5 ml
½ cup	125 ml
¾ cup	187.5 ml
1 cup	250 ml

Weight Conversion Measurements	
U.S.	**Metric**
1 ounce	28.4 g
8 ounces	227.5 g
16 ounces (1 pound)	455 g

Temperature Conversions

We've also included the following table and calculations so you can easily convert cooking temperatures for our recipes.

Cooking Temperature Conversions	
Celsius/Centigrade	0°C and 100°C are arbitrarily placed at the melting and boiling points of water and standard to the metric system
Fahrenheit	Fahrenheit established 0°F as the stabilized temperature when equal amounts of ice, water, and salt are mixed.

To convert temperatures in Fahrenheit to Celsius, use this formula:

$$C = (F - 32) \times 0.5555$$

So, for example, if you are baking at 350°F and want to know that temperature in Celsius, use this calculation:

$$C = (350 - 32) \times 0.5555 = 176.66°C$$

Selected References

Chapter 1: Cholesterol: A Key Factor in the Development of Heart Disease

Ajani, U. A., E. S. Ford, and A. H. Mokdad. "Dietary Fiber and C-Reactive Protein: Findings from National Health and Nutrition Examination Survey Data." *Journal of Nutrition* 134, no. 5 (May 2004): 1181–85.

Barghash, N. A., S. M. Elewa, E. A. Hamdi, A. A. Barghash, and R. El Dine. "Role of Plasma Homocysteine and Lipoprotein (a) in Coronary Artery Disease." *British Journal of Biomedical Science* 61, no. 2 (2004): 78–83.

Centers for Disease Control and Prevention. *Centers for Disease Control and Prevention: Diabetes Surveillance Report, 1999.* Atlanta: U.S. Department of Health and Human Services, 1999.

Christen, W. G., U. A. Ajani, R. J. Glynn, and C. H. Hennekens. "Blood Levels of Homocysteine and Increased Risks of Cardiovascular Disease: Causal or Casual?" *Archives of Internal Medicine* 160 (2000): 422–34.

de Maat, M. P., and A. Trion. "C-Reactive Protein as a Risk Factor Versus Risk Marker." *Current Opinion in Lipidology* 15, no. 6 (December 2004): 651–57.

Duvall, W. L. "Endothelial Dysfunction and Antioxidants." *Mt. Sinai Journal of Medicine* 72, no. 2 (March 2005): 71–80.

Ford, E. S., A. H. Mokdad, and S. Liu. "Healthy Eating Index and C-Reactive Protein Concentration: Findings from the National Health and Nutrition Examination Survey III, 1988–1994." *European Journal of Clinical Nutrition* 59, no. 2 (February 2005): 278–83.

Gao, X., O. I. Bermudez, and K. L. Tucker. "Plasma C-Reactive Protein and Homocysteine Concentrations Are Related to Frequent Fruit and Vegetable Intake in Hispanic and Non-Hispanic White Elders." *Journal of Nutrition* 134, no. 4 (April 2004): 913–18.

Geisel, J., B. Hennen, U. Hubner, J. P. Knapp, and W. Herrmann. "The Impact of Hyperhomocysteinemia as a Cardiovascular Risk Factor in the Prediction of Coronary Heart Disease." *Clinical Chemistry Laboratory Medicine* 41, no. 11 (November 2003): 1513–17.

Gerhard, G. T., and P. B. Duell. "Homocysteine and Atherosclerosis." *Current Opinion in Lipidology* 10 (1999): 417–28.

Grundy, S. M., I. J. Benjamin, G. L. Burke, et al. "Diabetes and Cardiovascular Disease: A Statement for Healthcare Professionals from the American Heart Association." *Circulation* 100 (1999): 1134–46.

Gu, K., C. C. Cowie, and M. I. Harris. "Diabetes and Decline in Heart Disease Mortality in US Adults." *JAMA* 281 (1999): 1291–97.

Juhan-Vague, I., M. C. Alessi, and P. Vague. "Thrombogenic and Fibrinolytic Factors and Cardiovascular Risk in Non-Insulin-Dependent Diabetes Mellitus." *Annals of Medicine* 28 (1996): 371–80.

Kelley, G. A., K. S. Kelley, and Z. Vu Tran. "Aerobic Exercise, Lipids and Lipoproteins in Overweight and Obese Adults: A Meta-Analysis of Randomized Controlled Trials." *International Journal of Obesity and Related Metabolic Disorders* 29, no. 8 (August 2005): 881–93.

Kullo, I. J., and C. M. Ballantyne. "Conditional Risk Factors for Atherosclerosis." *Mayo Clinic Proceedings* 80, no. 2 (February 2005): 219–30.

Malinow, M. R., A. G. Bostom, and R. M. Krauss. "Homocyst(e)ine, Diet, and Cardiovascular Diseases: A Statement for Healthcare Professionals from the Nutrition Committee, American Heart Association." *Circulation* 99 (1999): 178–82.

Rifai, N., J. Ma, F. M. Sacks, P. M. Ridker, W. J. Hernandez, M. J. Stampfer, and S. M. Marcovina. "Apolipoprotein(a) Size and Lipoprotein(a) Concentration and Future Risk of Angina Pectoris with Evidence of Severe Coronary Atherosclerosis in Men: The Physicians' Health Study." *Clinical Chemistry* 50, no. 8 (August 2004): 1364–71.

Schaefer, E. J. "Lipoproteins, Nutrition, and Heart Disease." *American Journal of Clinical Nutrition* 75, no. 2 (February 2002): 191–212.

Shai, I., E. B. Rimm, S. E. Hankinson, C. Cannuscio, G. Curhan, J. E. Manson, N. Rifai, M. J. Stampfer, and J. Ma. "Lipoprotein (a) and Coronary Heart Disease Among Women: Beyond a Cholesterol Carrier?" *European Heart Journal* 26 (August 2005): 1633–39.

Shai, I., M. J. Stampfer, J. Ma, J. E. Manson, S. E. Hankinson, C. Cannuscio, J. Selhub, G. Curhan, and E. B. Rimm. "Homocysteine as a Risk Factor for Coronary Heart Diseases and Its Association with Inflammatory Biomarkers, Lipids and Dietary Factors." *Atherosclerosis* 177, no. 2 (December 2004): 375–81.

Stocker, R., and J. F. Keaney Jr. "Role of Oxidative Modifications in Atherosclerosis." *Physiological Review* 84, no. 4 (October 2004): 1381–478.

Tholstrup, T., and S. Samman. "Postprandial Lipoprotein(a) Is Affected Differently by Specific Individual Dietary Fatty Acids in Healthy Young Men." *Journal of Nutrition* 134, no. 10 (October 2004): 2550–55.

U.S. Department of Agriculture. Center for Nutrition Policy and Promotion. *2005 Dietary Guidelines for Americans.*

Vrentzos, G., J. A. Papadakis, N. Malliaraki, E. A. Zacharis, K. Katsogridakis, A. N. Margioris, P. E. Vardas, and E. S. Ganotakis. "Association of Serum Total Homocysteine with the Extent of Ischemic Heart Disease in a Mediterranean Cohort." *Angiology* 55, no. 5 (September–October 2004): 517–24.

Weise, S. D., P. W. Grandjean, J. J. Rohack, J. W. Womack, and S. F. Crouse. "Acute Changes in Blood Lipids and Enzymes in Postmenopausal Women After Exercise." *Journal of Applied Physiology* 99, no. 2 (August 2005): 609–15.

Welch, G. N., and J. Loscalzo. "Homocysteine and Atherothrombosis." *New England Journal of Medicine* 338 (1998): 1042–50.

Wingard, D. L., and E. Barrett-Connor. "Heart Disease and Diabetes." In *Diabetes in America*, ed. National Diabetes Data Group. Washington, D.C.: National Institutes of Health, NIDDK, NIH publication no. 95-1468, 1995.

Zieske, A. W., R. P. Tracy, C. A. McMahan, E. E. Herderick, S. Homma, G. T. Malcom, H. C. McGill Jr., and J. P. Strong. "Elevated Serum C-Reactive Protein Levels and Advanced Atherosclerosis in Youth." *Arteriosclerosis, Thrombosis, and Vascular Biology* 25, no. 6 (June 2005): 1237–43.

Chapter 2: Focusing on Cholesterol: What the Numbers Mean

Baer, D. J., J. T. Judd, B. A. Clevidence, and R. P. Tracy. "Dietary Fatty Acids Affect Plasma Markers of Inflammation in Healthy Men Fed Controlled Diets: A Randomized Crossover Study." *American Journal of Clinical Nutrition* 79, no. 6 (June 2004): 969–73.

Barter, P. "HDL: A Recipe for Longevity." *Atherosclerosis Supplement* 5, no. 2 (May 2004): 25–31.

Brand-Miller, J. C. "Glycemic Index in Relation to Coronary Disease." *Asia Pacific Journal of Clinical Nutrition Supplement* 13 (2004): S3.

Brown, L., B. Rosner, W. C. Willett, and F. M. Sacks. "Cholesterol-Lowering Effects of Dietary Fiber: A Meta-Analysis." *American Journal of Clinical Nutrition* 69 (1999): 30–42.

National Institutes of Health, National Heart, Lung, and Blood Institute. National Cholesterol Education Program. "High Blood Cholesterol: What You Need to Know." (website).

von Eckardstein, A., M. Hersberger, and L. Rohrer. "Current Understanding of the Metabolism and Biological Actions of HDL." *Cur-*

rent Opinion in Clinical Nutrition and Metabolic Care 8, no. 2 (March 2005): 147–52.

Wierzbicki, A. S. "Have We Forgotten the Pivotal Role of High-Density Lipoprotein Cholesterol in Atherosclerosis Prevention?" *Current Medical Research and Opinion* 21, no. 2 (February 2005): 299–306.

Chapter 3: Fats, Carbs, and Your Cholesterol

Anderson, J. W., and S. R. Bridges. "Dietary Fiber Content of Selected Foods." *American Journal of Clinical Nutrition* 47 (1988): 440–47.

Anderson, J. W., and T. J. Hanna. "Impact of Nondigestible Carbohydrates on Serum Lipoproteins and Risk for Cardiovascular Disease." *Journal of Nutrition* 129, supplement 7 (1999): 1457S–1466S.

Bowes, A. D. *Bowes and Church's Food Values or Portions Commonly Used.* 14th edition. New York: Harper & Row, 1985.

Dickinson, S., and J. Brand-Miller. "Glycemic Index, Postprandial Glycemia and Cardiovascular Disease." *Current Opinion in Lipidology* 16, no. 1 (February 2005): 69–75.

Ford, E., and S. Liu. "Glycemic Index and Serum High-Density Lipoprotein Cholesterol Concentration Among U.S. Adults" *Archives of Internal Medicine* 161 (2001): 572–76.

Frost, G., A. A. Leeds, C. J. Dore, S. Madeiros, S. Brading, and A. Dornhorst. "Glycaemic Index as a Determinant of Serum HDL-Cholesterol Concentration." *Lancet* 353, no. 9158 (March 27, 1999): 1045–48.

Fung, T. T., F. B. Hu, M. A. Pereira, et al. "Whole-Grain Intake and the Risk of Type 2 Diabetes: A Prospective Study in Men." *American Journal of Clinical Nutrition* 76 (2002): 535–40.

Hu, F. B., E. Cho, K. M. Rexrode, C. M. Albert, and J. E. Manson. "Fish and Long-Chain Omega-3 Fatty Acid Intake and Risk of Coronary Heart Disease and Total Mortality in Diabetic Women." *Circulation* 107, no. 14 (April 15, 2003): 1852–57.

Jalili, T., R. E. C. Wildman, and D. M. Medeiros. "Nutraceutical Roles of Dietary Fiber." *Journal of Nutraceuticals, Functional, and Medical Foods* 2, no. 4 (2000): 19–34.

Khor, G. L. "Dietary Fat Quality: A Nutritional Epidemiologist's View." *Asia Pacific Journal of Clinical Nutrition* Supplement 13 (August 2004): S22.

King, D. E., B. M. Egan, and M. E. Geesey. "Relation of Dietary Fat and Fiber to Elevation of C-Reactive Protein." *American Journal of Cardiology* 92, no. 11 (December 1, 2003): 1335–39.

Knekt, P., J. Kumpulainen, R. Jarvinen, H. Rissanen, M. Heliovaara, A. Reunanen, T. Hakulinen, and A. Aromaa. "Flavonoid Intake and Risk of Chronic Diseases." *American Journal of Clinical Nutrition* 76, no. 3 (September 2002): 560–68.

Knopp, R. H., H. R. Superko, M. Davidson, W. Insull, C. A. Dujovne, P. O. Kwiterovich, J. H. Zavoral, K. Graham, R. R. O'Connor, and D. A. Edelman. "Long-Term Blood Cholesterol-Lowering Effects of a Dietary Fiber Supplement." *American Journal of Preventive Medicine* 17, no. 1 (July 1999): 18–23.

Kris-Etherton, P. M., K. D. Hecker, and A. E. Binkoski. "Polyunsaturated Fatty Acids and Cardiovascular Health." *Nutrition Review* 62, no. 11 (November 2004): 414–26.

Lee, Y. H., and R. E. Pratley. "The Evolving Role of Inflammation in Obesity and the Metabolic Syndrome." *Current Diabetes Report* 5, no. 1 (February 2005): 70–75.

Lichtenstein, A. H., A. T. Erkkila, B. Lamarche, U. S. Schwab, S. M. Jalbert, and L. M. Ausman. "Influence of Hydrogenated Fat and Butter on CVD Risk Factors: Remnant-Like Particles, Glucose and Insulin, Blood Pressure and C-Reactive Protein." *Atherosclerosis* 171, no. 1 (November 2003): 97–107.

Liu, S., J. Manson, M. Stampfer, M. Holmes, F. Hu, S. Hankinson, and W. Willett. "Dietary Glycemic Load Assessed by Food-Frequency Questionnaire in Relation to Plasma High-Density-Lipoprotein Cholesterol and Fasting Plasma Triacylglycerols in

Postmenopausal Women." *American Journal of Clinical Nutrition* 73, no. 3 (March 2001), 560–66.

Liu, S., W. C. Willett, M. J. Stampfer, et al. "A Prospective Study of Dietary Glycemic Load, Carbohydrate Intake, and Risk of Coronary Heart Disease in U.S. Women." *American Journal of Clinical Nutrition* 71 (2001): 1455–61.

Lopez-Garcia, E., M. B. Schulze, J. B. Meigs, J. E. Manson, N. Rifai, M. J. Stampfer, W. C. Willett, and F. B. Hu. "Consumption of Trans Fatty Acids Is Related to Plasma Biomarkers of Inflammation and Endothelial Dysfunction." *Journal of Nutrition* 135, no. 3 (March 2005): 562–66.

Lopez-Garcia, E., M. B. Schulze, J. E. Manson, J. B. Meigs, C. M. Albert, N. Rifai, W. C. Willett, and F. B. Hu. "Consumption of (n-3) Fatty Acids Is Related to Plasma Biomarkers of Inflammation and Endothelial Activation in Women." *Journal of Nutrition* 134, no. 7 (July 2004): 1806–11.

Lopez-Garcia, E., M. B. Schulze, T. T. Fung, J. B. Meigs, N. Rifai, J. E. Manson, and F. B. Hu. "Major Dietary Patterns Are Related to Plasma Concentrations of Markers of Inflammation and Endothelial Dysfunction." *American Journal of Clinical Nutrition* 80, no. 4 (October 2004): 1029–35.

McKeown, N. M., J. B. Meigs, and S. Liu. "Carbohydrate Nutrition, Insulin Resistance, and the Prevalence of the Metabolic Syndrome in the Framingham Offspring Cohort." *Diabetes Care* 27 (2004): 538–46.

McKeown, N. M., J. B. Meigs, S. Liu, P. W. Wilson, and P. F. Jacques. "Whole-Grain Intake Is Favorably Associated with Metabolic Risk Factors for Type 2 Diabetes and Cardiovascular Disease in the Framingham Offspring Study." *American Journal of Clinical Nutrition* 76, no. 2 (August 2002): 390–98.

Mozaffarian, D., T. Pischon, S. E. Hankinson, N. Rifai, K. Joshipura, W. C. Willett, and E. B. Rimm. "Dietary Intake of Trans Fatty Acids and Systemic Inflammation in Women." *American Journal of Clinical Nutrition* 79, no. 4 (April 2004): 606–12.

National Cholesterol Education Program. *Third Report of the Expert Panel on Detection, Evaluation, and Treatment of High Blood Cholesterol in Adults (Adult Treatment Panel III)*. National Heart, Lung, and Blood Institute, National Institutes of Health: May 2001.

National Heart, Lung, and Blood Institute, National Institutes of Health.

National Institutes of Health, Office of Dietary Supplements.

Oh, K., F. B. Hu, J. E. Manson, M. J. Stampfer, and W. C. Willett. "Dietary Fat Intake and Risk of Coronary Heart Disease in Women: 20 Years of Follow-Up of the Nurses' Health Study." *American Journal of Epidemiology* 161, no. 7 (April 1, 2005): 672–79.

Pereira, M. A., E. O'Reilly, K. Augustsson, et al. "Dietary Fiber and Risk of Coronary Heart Disease: A Pooled Analysis of Cohort Studies." *Archives of Internal Medicine* 164 (2004): 370–76.

Pereira, M. A., J. Swain, A. B. Goldfine, N. Rifai, and D. S. Ludwig. "Effects of a Low-Glycemic Load Diet on Resting Energy Expenditure and Heart Disease Risk Factors During Weight Loss." *JAMA* 292, no. 20 (November 24, 2004): 2482–90.

Rimm, E. B., A. Ascherio, E. Giovannucci, D. Spiegelman, M. J. Stampfer, and W. C. Willett. "Vegetable, Fruit, and Cereal Fiber Intake and Risk of Coronary Heart Disease Among Men." *JAMA* 275 (1996): 447–51.

Schulze, M. B., S. Liu, E. B. Rimm, J. E. Manson, W. C. Willett, and F. B. Hu. "Glycemic Index, Glycemic Load, and Dietary Fiber Intake and Incidence of Type 2 Diabetes in Younger and Middle-Aged Women." *American Journal of Clinical Nutrition* 80 (2004): 348–56.

Tholstrup, T., and S. Samman. "Postprandial Lipoprotein(a) Is Affected Differently by Specific Individual Dietary Fatty Acids in Healthy Young Men." *Journal of Nutrition* 134, no. 10 (October 2004): 2550–55.

van Herpen-Broekmans, W. M., I. A. Klopping-Ketelaars, M. L. Bots, C. Kluft, H. Princen, H. F. Hendriks, L. B. Tijburg, G. van Poppel, and A. F. Kardinaal. "Serum Carotenoids and Vitamins in Relation to Markers of Endothelial Function and Inflammation." *European Journal of Epidemiology* 19, no. 10 (2004): 915–21.

Van Horn, L. "Fiber, Lipids, and Coronary Heart Disease. A Statement for Healthcare Professionals from the Nutrition Committee, American Heart Association." *Circulation* 95 (1997): 2701–4.

Wolf, A., J. E. Manson, M. J. Stampfer, et al. "Long-Term Intake of Dietary Fiber and Decreased Risk of Coronary Heart Disease Among Women." *JAMA* 281 (1999): 1998–2004.

Chapter 4: Antioxidants, Phytyonutrients, and Other Cholesterol-Lowering Nutrients

Andersson, T. L., J. Matz, G. A. Ferns, and E. E. Anggard. "Vitamin E Reverses Cholesterol-Induced Endothelial Dysfunction in the Rabbit Coronary Circulation." *Atherosclerosis* 111 (1994): 39–45.

Arai, Y., S. Watanabe, M. Kimira, K. Shimoi, R. Mochizuki, and N. Kinae. "Dietary Intakes of Flavonols, Flavones, and Isoflavones by Japanese Women and the Inverse Correlation Between Quercetin Intake and Plasma LDL Cholesterol Concentration." *Journal of Nutrition* 130, no. 9 (September 2000): 2243–50.

Auger, C., P. L. Teissedre, P. Gerain, N. Lequeux, A. Bornet, S. Serisier, P. Besancon, B. Caporiccio, J. P. Cristol, and J. M. Rouanet. "Dietary Wine Phenolics Catechin, Quercetin, and Resveratrol Efficiently Protect Hypercholesterolemic Hamsters Against Aortic Fatty Streak Accumulation." *Journal of Agriculture and Food Chemistry* 53, no. 6 (March 23, 2005): 2015–21.

Bok, S. H., S. Y. Park, Y. B. Park, M. K. Lee, S. M. Jeon, T. S. Jeong, and M. S. Choi. "Quercetin Dihydrate and Gallate Supplements Lower Plasma and Hepatic Lipids and Change Activities of Hepatic Antioxidant Enzymes in High Cholesterol-Fed Rats." *International Journal for Vitamin and Nutrition Research* 72, no. 3 (May 2002): 161–69.

Bordia, A., S. K. Verma, and K. C. Srivastava. "Effect of Garlic (*Allium Sativum*) on Blood Lipids, Blood Sugar, Fibrinogen and Fibrinolytic

Activity in Patients with Coronary Artery Disease." *Prostaglandins, Leukotrienes, and Essential Fatty Acids* 58, no. 4 (April 1998): 257–63.

Brown, L., E. B. Rimm, J. M. Seddon, E. L. Giovannucci, L. Chasan-Taber, D. Spiegelman, W. C. Willett, and S. E. Hankinson. "A Prospective Study of Carotenoid Intake and Risk of Cataract Extraction in U.S. Men." *American Journal of Clinical Nutrition* 70, no. 4 (October 1999): 517–24.

Centers for Disease Control and Prevention. *Centers for Disease Control and Prevention: Diabetes Surveillance Report, 1999.* Atlanta: U.S. Department of Health and Human Services, 1999.

Clifton, P. M., M. Noakes, D. Ross, A. Fassoulakis, M. Cehun, and P. Nestel. "High Dietary Intake of Phytosterol Esters Decreases Carotenoids and Increases Plasma Plant Sterol Levels with No Additional Cholesterol Lowering." *Journal of Lipid Research* 45, no. 8 (August 2004): 1493–99.

Colgan, H. A., S. Floyd, E. J. Noone, M. J. Gibney, and H. M. Roche. "Increased Intake of Fruit and Vegetables and a Low-Fat Diet, with and Without Low-Fat Plant Sterol-Enriched Spread Consumption: Effects on Plasma Lipoprotein and Carotenoid Metabolism." *Journal of Human Nutrition and Dietetics* 17, no. 6 (December 2004): 561–79; quiz 571–74.

Cooper, D. "Carotenoids in Health and Disease: Recent Scientific Evaluations, Research Recommendations and the Consumer Supplement: Proceedings of Symposium to Honor the Memory of James Allen Olson." *Journal of Nutrition* 134 (January 2004): 221S–224S.

Exner, M., M. Hermann, R. Hofbauer, et al. "Genistein Prevents the Glucose Autooxidation Mediated Atherogenic Modification of Low Density Lipoprotein." *Free Radical Research* 34, no. 1 (January 2001): 101–12.

Ferri, N., K. Yokoyama, M. Sadilek, R. Paoletti, R. Apitz-Castro, M. H. Gelb, and A. Corsini. "Ajoene, a Garlic Compound, Inhibits Protein Prenylation and Arterial Smooth Muscle Cell Proliferation." *British Journal of Pharmacology* 138, no. 5 (March 2003): 811–18.

Grundy, S. M., I. J. Benjamin, G. L. Burke, et al. "Diabetes and Cardiovascular Disease: A Statement for Healthcare Professionals from the American Heart Association." *Circulation* 100 (1999): 1134–46.

Haffner, S. M., S. Lehto, T. Ronnemaa, K. Pyorala, and M. Laakso. "Mortality from Coronary Heart Disease in Subjects with Type 2 Diabetes and in Nondiabetic Subjects with and Without Prior Myocardial Infarction." *New England Journal of Medicine* 339 (1998): 229–34.

Heber, D. "Vegetables, Fruits and Phytoestrogens in the Prevention of Diseases." *Journal of Postgraduate Medicine* 50, no. 2 (April–June 2004): 145–49.

Heber, D., and S. Bowerman. "Applying Science to Changing Dietary Patterns." *Journal of Nutrition* 131 (November 2001): 3078S–3081S.

Hertog, M. G., E. J. Feskens, P. C. Hollman, M. B. Katan, and D. Kromhout. "Dietary Antioxidant Flavonoids and Risk of Coronary Heart Disease: The Zutphen Elderly Study." *Lancet* 342, no. 8878 (October 23, 1993): 1007–11.

Jeon, S. M., Y. B. Park, and M. S. Choi. "Antihypercholesterolemic Property of Naringin Alters Plasma and Tissue Lipids, Cholesterol-Regulating Enzymes, Fecal Sterol and Tissue Morphology in Rabbits." *Clinical Nutrition* 23, no. 5 (October 2004): 1025–34.

Kamada, C., E. L. da Silva, M. Ohnishi-Kameyama, J. H. Moon, and J. Terao. "Attenuation of Lipid Peroxidation and Hyperlipidemia by Quercetin Glucoside in the Aorta of High Cholesterol-Fed Rabbit." *Free Radical Research* 39, no. 2 (February 2005): 185–94.

Kamal-Eldin, A., J. Frank, A. Razdan, S. Tengblad, S. Basu, and B. Vessby. "Effects of Dietary Phenolic Compounds on Tocopherol, Cholesterol, and Fatty Acids in Rats." *Lipids* 35, no. 4 (April 2000): 427–35.

Kim, H. J., G. T. Oh, Y. B. Park, M. K. Lee, H. J. Seo, and M. S. Choi. "Naringin Alters the Cholesterol Biosynthesis and Antioxidant Enzyme Activities in LDL Receptor-Knockout Mice Under Cholesterol Fed Condition." *Life Science* 74, no. 13 (February 13, 2004): 1621–34.

Knekt, P., J. Kumpulainen, R. Jarvinen, H. Rissanen, M. Heliovaara, A. Reunanen, T. Hakulinen, and A. Aromaa. "Flavonoid Intake and Risk of Chronic Diseases." *American Journal of Clinical Nutrition* 76, no. 3 (September 2002): 560–68.

Knekt, P., J. Ritz, M. A. Pereira, E. J. O'Reilly, K. Augustsson, G. E. Fraser, U. Goldbourt, B. L. Heitmann, G. Hallmans, S. Liu, P. Pietinen, D. Spiegelman, J. Stevens, J. Virtamo, W. C. Willett, E. B. Rimm, and A. Ascherio. "Antioxidant Vitamins and Coronary Heart Disease Risk: A Pooled Analysis of 9 Cohorts." *American Journal of Clinical Nutrition* 80, no. 6 (December 2004): 1508–20.

Kromhout, D. "Fatty Acids, Antioxidants, and Coronary Heart Disease from an Epidemiological Perspective." *Lipids* Supplement 34 (1999): S27–31.

Kurowska, E. M., and J. A. Manthey. "Hypolipidemic Effects and Absorption of Citrus Polymethoxylated Flavones in Hamsters with Diet-Induced Hypercholesterolemia." *Journal of Agriculture and Food Chemistry* 52, no. 10 (May 19, 2004): 2879–86.

Lissin, L.W., and J. P. Cooke. "Phytoestrogens and Cardiovascular Health." *Journal of the American College of Cardiology* 35, no. 6 (May 2000): 1403–10.

Liu, R. H. "Health Benefits of Fruits and Vegetables Are from Additive and Synergistic Combination of Phytochemicals." *American Journal of Clinical Nutrition* 78 (2003): 517S–520S.

Liu, S., W. C. Willett, M. J. Stampfer, et al. "A Prospective Study of Dietary Glycemic Load, Carbohydrate Intake and Risk of Coronary Heart Disease in U.S. Women." *American Journal of Clinical Nutrition* 71 (2000): 1455–61.

Manson, J. E., J. M. Gaziano, A. Spelsberg, et al. "A Secondary Prevention Trial of Antioxidant Vitamins and Cardiovascular Disease in Women. Rationale, Design, and Methods. The WACS Research Group." *Annals of Epidemiology* 5 (1995): 261–69.

Maron, D. J. "Flavonoids for Reduction of Atherosclerotic Risk." *Current Atherosclerosis* Report 6, no. 1 (January 2004): 73–78.

McDermott, J. H. "Antioxidant Nutrients: Current Dietary Recommendations and Research Update." *Journal of the American Pharmacology Association (Wash)* 40, no. 6 (November–December 2000): 785–99.

Miura, D., Y. Miura, and K. Yagasaki. "Hypolipidemic Action of Dietary Resveratrol, a Phytoalexin in Grapes and Red Wine, in Hepatoma-Bearing Rats." *Life Science* 73, no. 11 (August 1, 2003): 1393–400.

Miwa, Y., M. Yamada, T. Sunayama, H. Mitsuzumi, Y. Tsuzaki, H. Chaen, Y. Mishima, and M. Kibata. "Effects of Glucosyl Hesperidin on Serum Lipids in Hyperlipidemic Subjects: Preferential Reduction in Elevated Serum Triglyceride Level." *Journal of Nutritional Science and Vitaminology (Tokyo)* 50, no. 3 (June 2004): 211–18.

National Institute on Aging Age Page. "Life Extension: Science or Science Fiction?" U.S. Department of Health and Human Services, Public Health Service, National Institutes of Health.

NCI, 5-a-Day Website, "Glossary of Phytochemicals." 5aday.gov.

NIA Research Goal B: Understand Healthy Aging Processes Subgoal 1: Unlock the Secrets of Aging, Health, and Longevity.

Osganian, S. K., M. J. Stampfer, E. Rimm, D. Spiegelman, J. E. Manson, and W. C. Willett. "Dietary Carotenoids and Risk of Coronary Artery Disease in Women." *American Journal of Clinical Nutrition* 77, no. 6 (June 2003): 1390–99.

Ou, C. C., S. M. Tsao, M. C. Lin, and M. C. Yin. "Protective Action on Human LDL Against Oxidation and Glycation by Four Organosulfur Compounds Derived from Garlic." *Lipids* 38, no. 3 (March 2003): 219–24.

Rao, A. V. "Lycopene, Tomatoes, and the Prevention of Coronary Heart Disease." *Experimental Biology and Medicine (Maywood)* 227, no. 10 (November 2002): 908–13.

Reed, J. "Cranberry Flavonoids, Atherosclerosis and Cardiovascular Health." *Critical Reviews of Food Science and Nutrition* Supplement 42, no. 3 (2002): 301–16.

Ribaya-Mercado, J. D., and J. B. Blumberg. "Lutein and Zeaxanthin and Their Potential Roles in Disease Prevention." *Journal of the American College of Nutrition* Supplement 23, no. 6 (December 2004): 567S–587S.

Rimm, E. B., and M. J. Stampfer. "Antioxidants for Vascular Disease." *Medical Clinics of North America* 84 (2000): 239–49.

Rimm, E. B., M. J. Stampfer, A. Ascherio, E. Giovannucci, G. A. Colditz, and W. C. Willett. "Vitamin E Consumption and the Risk of Coronary Heart Disease in Men." *New England Journal of Medicine* 328 (1993): 1450–56.

Rissanen, T., S. Voutilainen, K. Nyyssonen, and J. T. Salonen. "Lycopene, Atherosclerosis, and Coronary Heart Disease." *Experimental Biology and Medicine (Maywood)* 227, no. 10 (November 2002): 900–907.

Rissanen, T. H., S. Voutilainen, K. Nyyssonen, R. Salonen, G. A. Kaplan, and J. T. Salonen. "Serum Lycopene Concentrations and Carotid Atherosclerosis: The Kuopio Ischaemic Heart Disease Risk Factor Study." *American Journal of Clinical Nutrition* 77, no. 1 (January 2003): 133–8.

Sanchez-Moreno, C., G. Cao, B. Ou, and R. L. Prior. "Anthocyanin and Proanthocyanidin Content in Selected White and Red Wines. Oxygen Radical Absorbance Capacity Comparison with Nontraditional Wines Obtained from Highbush Blueberry." *Journal of Agriculture and Food Chemistry* 51, no. 17 (August 13, 2003): 4889–96.

Spence, J. D., V. J. Howard, L. E. Chambless, et al. "Vitamin Intervention for Stroke Prevention (VISP) Trial: Rationale and Design." *Neuroepidemiology* 20 (2001): 16–25.

Stampfer, M. J., C. H. Hennekens, J. E. Manson, G. A. Colditz, B. Rosner, and W. C. Willett. "Vitamin E Consumption and the Risk of Coronary Disease in Women." *New England Journal of Medicine* 328 (1993): 1444–49.

Tijburg, L. B. M., T. Mattern, J. D. Folts, U. M. Weisgerber, and M. B. Katan. "Tea Flavonoids and Cardiovascular Diseases: A Review." *Critical Review of Food Science and Nutrition* 37 (1997): 771–85.

Ting, H. H., F. K. Timimi, K. S. Boles, S. J. Creager, P. Ganz, and M. A. Creager. "Vitamin C Improves Endothelium-Dependent Vasodilation in Patients with Non-Insulin-Dependent Diabetes Mellitus." *Journal of Clinical Investigation* 97 (1996): 22–28.

United States Department of Agriculture, Agricultural Research Service. *Food and Nutrient Intakes by Individuals in the United States, by Sex and Age, 1994–1996.* Nationwide Food Surveys Report No. 96–2. Washington, D.C.: USDA, 1998.

van der Schouw, Y. T., L. Sampson, W. C. Willett, and E. B. Rimm. "The Usual Intake of Lignans but Not That of Isoflavones May Be Related to Cardiovascular Risk Factors in U.S. Men." *Journal of Nutrition* 135, no. 2 (February 2005): 260–66.

Vaskonen, T. "Dietary Minerals and Modification of Cardiovascular Risk Factors." *Journal of Nutritional Biochemistry* 14, no. 9 (September 2003): 492–506.

Vinson, J. A., and J. Jang. "In Vitro and In Vivo Lipoprotein Antioxidant Effect of a Citrus Extract and Ascorbic Acid on Normal and Hypercholesterolemic Human Subjects." *Journal of Medicinal Food* 4, no. 4 (Winter 2001): 187–92.

Wan, Y., J. A. Vinson, T. D. Etherton, J. Proch, S. A. Lazarus, and P. M. Kris-Etherton. "Effects of Cocoa Powder and Dark Chocolate on LDL Oxidative Susceptibility and Prostaglandin Concentrations in Humans." *American Journal of Clinical Nutrition* 74, no. 5 (November 2001): 596–602.

Weisburger, J. H. "Chemopreventive Effects of Cocoa Polyphenols on Chronic Diseases." *Experimental Biology and Medicine (Maywood)* 226, no. 10 (November 2001): 891–97.

Whitman, S. C., E. M. Kurowska, J. A. Manthey, and A. Daugherty. "Nobiletin, a Citrus Flavonoid Isolated from Tangerines, Selectively Inhibits Class A Scavenger Receptor-Mediated Metabolism of Acetylated LDL by Mouse Macrophages." *Atherosclerosis* 178, no. 1 (January 2005): 25–32.

Woodman, O. L., and E. C. Chan. "Vascular and Anti-Oxidant Actions of Flavonols and Flavones." *Clinical and Experimental Pharmacology and Physiology* 31, no. 11 (November 2004): 786–90.

Wu, X., G. Beecher, J. Holden, D. Haytowitz, S. Gebhardt, and R. Prior. "Lipophilic and Hydrophilic Antioxident Capacities of Common Foods in the United States." *Journal of Agricultural and Food Chemistry* 52 (2004): 4026–37.

Yao, L. H., Y. M. Jiang, J. Shi, F. A. Tomas-Barberan, N. Datta, R. Singanusong, and S. S. Chen. "Flavonoids in Food and Their Health Benefits." *Plant Foods for Human Nutrition* 59, no. 3 (Summer 2004): 113–22.

Yusuf, S., G. Dagenais, J. Pogue, J. Bosch, and P. Sleight. "Vitamin E Supplementation and Cardiovascular Events in High-Risk Patients. The Heart Outcomes Prevention Evaluation Study Investigators." *New England Journal of Medicine* 342 (2000): 154–60.

Chapter 5: Cholesterol-Lowering Foods

Adom, K. K., and R. H. Liu. "Antioxidant Activity of Grains." *Journal of Agriculture and Food Chemistry* 50 (2002): 6182–87.

Adom, K. K., M. E. Sorrells, and R. H. Liu. "Phytochemicals and Antioxidant Activity of Wheat Varieties." *Journal of Agriculture and Food Chemistry* 51 (2003): 7825–34.

Ali, A. A., M. T. Velasquez, C. T. Hansen, A. I. Mohamed, and S. J. Bhathena. "Effects of Soybean Isoflavones, Probiotics, and Their Interactions on Lipid Metabolism and Endocrine System in an Animal Model of Obesity and Diabetes." *Journal of Nutritional and Biochemistry* 15, no. 10 (October 2004): 583–90.

The Alpha-Tocopherol, Beta Carotene Cancer Prevention Study Group. "The Effect of Vitamin E and ß-Carotene on the Incidence of Lung Cancer and Other Cancers in Male Smokers." *New England Journal of Medicine* 330 (1994): 1029–35.

Andrikopoulos, N. K., A. C. Kaliora, A. N. Assimopoulou, and V. P. Papageorgiou. "Inhibitory Activity of Minor Polyphenolic and Non-polyphenolic Constituents of Olive Oil Against in Vitro Low-Density Lipoprotein Oxidation." *Journal of Medicinal Food* 5, no. 1 (Spring 2002): 1–7.

Appel, L. J., T. J. Moore, E. Obarzanek, et al. "A Clinical Trial of the Effects of Dietary Patterns on Blood Pressure. DASH Collaborative Research Group." *New England Journal of Medicine* 336 (1997): 1117–24.

Auger, C., P. L. Teissedre, P. Gerain, N. Lequeux, A. Bornet, S. Serisier, P. Besancon, B. Caporiccio, J. P. Cristol, and J. M. Rouanet. "Dietary Wine Phenolics Catechin, Quercetin, and Resveratrol Efficiently Protect Hypercholesterolemic Hamsters Against Aortic Fatty Streak Accumulation." *Journal of Agriculture and Food Chemistry* 53, no. 6 (March 23, 2005): 2015–21.

Aviram, M., M. Rosenblat, D. Gaitini, S. Nitecki, A. Hoffman, L. Dornfeld, N. Volkova, D. Presser, J. Attias, H. Liker, and T. Hayek. "Pomegranate Juice Consumption for 3 Years by Patients with Carotid Artery Stenosis Reduces Common Carotid Intima-Media Thickness, Blood Pressure and LDL Oxidation." *Clinical Nutrition* 23, no. 3 (June 2004): 423–33.

Behall, K. M., D. J. Scholfield, and J. Hallfrisch. "Diets Containing Barley Significantly Reduce Lipids in Mildly Hypercholesterolemic Men and Women." *American Journal of Clinical Nutrition* 80, no. 5 (November 2004): 1185–93.

Bloedon, L. T., and P. O. Szapary. "Flaxseed and Cardiovascular Risk." *Nutrition Review* 62, no. 1 (January 2004): 18–27.

Blot, W. J., J. Y. Li, P. R. Taylor, W. Guo, S. Dawsey, G. Q. Wang, C. S. Yang, S. F. Zheng, M. Gail, et al. "Nutrition Intervention Trials in Linxian, China: Supplementation with Specific Vitamin/Mineral Combinations, Cancer Incidence, and Disease-Specific Mortality in the General Population." *Journal of the National Cancer Institute* 85 (1993): 1483–92.

Bruce, B., G. A. Spiller, L. M. Klevay, and S. K. Gallagher. "A Diet High in Whole and Unrefined Foods Favorably Alters Lipids, Antioxidant Defenses, and Colon Function." *Journal of the American College of Nutrition* 19, no. 1 (February 2000): 61–67.

Colgan, H. A., S. Floyd, E. J. Noone, M. J. Gibney, and H. M. Roche. "Increased Intake of Fruit and Vegetables and a Low-Fat Diet, with and Without Low-Fat Plant Sterol-Enriched Spread Consumption: Effects on Plasma Lipoprotein and Carotenoid Metabolism." *Journal of Human Nutrition and Dietetics* 17, no. 6 (December 2004): 561–69; quiz 571–74.

Czerwinski, J., E. Bartnikowska, H. Leontowicz, E. Lange, M. Leontowicz, E. Katrich, S. Trakhtenberg, and S. Gorinstein. "Oat (*Avena Sativa L.*) and Amaranth (*Amaranthus Hypochondriacus*) Meals Positively Affect Plasma Lipid Profile in Rats Fed Cholesterol-Containing Diets." *Journal of Nutritional Biochemistry* 15, no. 10 (October 2004): 622–29.

Djousse, L., D. K. Arnett, H. Coon, M. A. Province, L. L. Moore, and R. C. Ellison. "Fruit and Vegetable Consumption and LDL Cholesterol: The National Heart, Lung, and Blood Institute Family Heart Study." *American Journal of Clinical Nutrition* 79 (2004): 213–17.

Eberhardt, M. V., C. Y. Lee, and R. H. Liu. "Antioxidant Activity of Fresh Apples." *Nature* 405 (2000): 903–4.

Engelman, H. M., D. L. Alekel, L. N. Hanson, A. G. Kanthasamy, and M. B. Reddy. "Blood Lipid and Oxidative Stress Responses to Soy Protein with Isoflavones and Phytic Acid in Postmenopausal Women." *American Journal of Clinical Nutrition* 81, no. 3 (March 2005): 590–96.

Erba, D., P. Riso, A. Bordoni, P. Foti, P. L. Biagi, and G. Testolin. "Effectiveness of Moderate Green Tea Consumption on Antioxidative Status and Plasma Lipid Profile in Humans." *Journal of Nutritional Biochemistry* 16, no. 3 (March 2005): 144–49.

Erdman, J., for the AHA Nutrition Committee. "Soy Protein and Cardiovascular Disease: A Statement for Healthcare Professionals from the Nutrition Committee of the AHA." *Circulation* 102 (2000): 2555.

Gebhardt, R. "Inhibition of Cholesterol Biosynthesis in Primary Cultured Rat Hepatocytes by Artichoke (*Cynara Scolymus L.*) Extracts." *Journal of Pharmacology and Experimental Therapeutics* 286, no. 3 (September 1998): 1122–28.

Greenberg, E. R., J. A. Baron, T. A. Stuckel, M. M. Stevens, and J. S. Mandel. "A Clinical Trial of ß-Carotene to Prevent Basal Cell and Squamous Cell Cancers of the Skin." *New England Journal of Medicine* 323 (1990): 789–95.

Heber, D. "Vegetables, Fruits and Phytoestrogens in the Prevention of Diseases." *Journal of Postgraduate Medicine* 50 (2004): 145–49.

Hennekens, C. H., J. E. Buring, J. E. Manson, M. Stampfer, and B. Rosner. "Lack of Effect of Long-Term Supplementation with ß-Carotene on the Incidence of Malignant Neoplasms and Cardiovascular Disease." *New England Journal of Medicine* 334 (1996): 1145–49.

Hung, H. C., K. J. Joshipura, R. Jiang, et al. "Fruit and Vegetable Intake and Risk of Major Chronic Disease." *Journal of the National Cancer Institute* 96 (2004): 1577–84.

Jacobs, D., and L. Steffen. "Nutrients, Foods and Dietary Patterns as Exposures in Research: A Framework for Food Synergy." *American Journal of Clinical Nutrition* Supplement 78, no. 3 (September 2003): 508S–513S.

Jambazian, P. R., E. Haddad, S. Rajaram, J. Tanzman, and J. Sabate. "Almonds in the Diet Simultaneously Improve Plasma Alpha-Tocopherol Concentrations and Reduce Plasma Lipids." *Journal of the American Dietetic Association* 105, no. 3 (March 2005): 449–54.

Jenkins, D. J., C. W. Kendall, A. Marchie, T. L. Parker, P. W. Connelly, W. Qian, J. S. Haight, D. Faulkner, E. Vidgen, K. G. Lapsley, and G. A. Spiller. "Dose Response of Almonds on Coronary Heart Disease Risk Factors: Blood Lipids, Oxidized Low-Density Lipoproteins, Lipoprotein(a), Homocysteine, and Pulmonary Nitric Oxide:

A Randomized, Controlled, Crossover Trial." *Circulation* 106, no. 11 (September 10, 2002): 1327–32.

Lewis, N., and J. Ruud. "Apples in the American Diet." *Nutrition and Clinical Care* 7, no. 2 (April–June 2004): 82–88.

Li, S. Q., and Q. H. Zhang. "Advances in the Development of Functional Foods from Buckwheat." *Critical Review of Food Science and Nutrition* 41, no. 6 (September 2001): 451–64.

Liu, R. H. "Health Benefits of Fruits and Vegetables Are from Additive and Synergistic Combination of Phytochemicals." *American Journal of Clinical Nutrition* 78 (2003): 517S–520S.

McKeown, N. M., J. B. Meigs, S. Liu, P. W. Wilson, and P. F. Jacques. "Whole-Grain Intake Is Favorably Associated with Metabolic Risk Factors for Type 2 Diabetes and Cardiovascular Disease in the Framingham Offspring Study." *American Journal of Clinical Nutrition* 76 (2002): 390–98.

Nicolle, C., N. Cardinault, O. Aprikian, J. Busserolles, P. Grolier, E. Rock, C. Demigne, A. Mazur, A. Scalbert, P. Amouroux, and C. Remesy. "Effect of Carrot Intake on Cholesterol Metabolism and on Antioxidant Status in Cholesterol-Fed Rat." *European Journal of Nutrition* 42, no. 5 (October 2003): 254–61.

Ommen, G. S., G. E. Goodman, M. D. Thomquist, J. Barnes, and M. R. Cullen. "Effects of a Combination of ß-Carotene and Vitamin A on Lung Cancer and Cardiovascular Disease." *New England Journal of Medicine* 334 (1996): 1150–55.

Prasad, K. "Hypocholesterolemic and Antiatherosclerotic Effect of Flax Lignan Complex Isolated from Flaxseed." *Atherosclerosis* 179, no. 2 (April 2005): 269–75.

Rao, A. V. "Lycopene, Tomatoes, and the Prevention of Coronary Heart Disease." *Experimental Biology and Medicine (Maywood)* 227, no. 10 (November 2002): 908–13.

Reed, J. "Cranberry Flavonoids, Atherosclerosis and Cardiovascular Health." *Critical Review of Food Science and Nutrition* Supplement 42, no. 3 (2002): 301–16.

Rimm, E. B., A. Ascherio, E. Giovannucci, D. Spiegelman, M. J. Stampfer, and W. C. Willett. "Vegetable, Fruit, and Cereal Fiber Intake and Risk of Coronary Heart Disease Among Men." *JAMA* 275 (1996): 447–51.

Salonen, J. T., K. Nyyssonen, R. Salonen, H. M. Lakka, J. Kaikkonen, E. Porkkala-Sarataho, S. Voutilainen, T. A. Lakka, and T. Rissanen, et al. "Antioxidant Supplementation in Atherosclerosis Prevention (ASAP) Study: A Randomized Trial of the Effect of Vitamins E and C on 3-Year Progression of Carotid Atherosclerosis." *Journal of Internal Medicine* 248 (2000): 377–86.

Slavin, J. "Why Whole Grains Are Protective: Biological Mechanisms." *Proceedings of the Nutrition Society* 62, no. 1 (February 2003): 129–34.

Stein, J. H., J. G. Keevil, D. A. Wiebe, S. Aeschlimann, and J. D. Folts. "Purple Grape Juice Improves Endothelial Function and Reduces the Susceptibility of LDL Cholesterol to Oxidation in Patients with Coronary Artery Disease." *Circulation* 100, no. 10 (September 7, 1999): 1050–55.

Stephens, N. G., A. Parsons, P. M. Schofield, F. Kelly, K. Cheeseman, and M. J. Mitchinson. "Randomized Controlled Trial of Vitamin E in Patients with Coronary Disease: Cambridge Heart Antioxidant Study (CHAOS)." *Lancet* 347 (1996): 781–86.

Tapsell, L. C., L. J. Gillen, C. S. Patch, M. Batterham, A. Owen, M. Bare, and M. Kennedy. "Including Walnuts in a Low-Fat/Modified-Fat Diet Improves HDL Cholesterol-to-Total Cholesterol Ratios in Patients with Type 2 Diabetes." *Diabetes Care* 27, no. 12 (December 2004): 2777–83.

Weisburger, J. H. "Chemopreventive Effects of Cocoa Polyphenols on Chronic Diseases." *Experimental Biology and Medicine (Maywood)* 226, no. 10 (November 2001): 891–97.

Yeh, Y. Y., and L. Liu. "Cholesterol-Lowering Effect of Garlic Extracts and Organosulfur Compounds: Human and Animal Studies." *Journal of Nutrition* 131, no. 3S (March 2001): 989S–993S.

Yusuf, S., G. Dagenais, J. Pogue, J. Bosch, and P. Sleight. "Vitamin E Supplementation and Cardiovascular Events in High-Risk Patients. The Heart Outcomes Prevention Evaluation Study Investigators." *New England Journal of Medicine* 342 (2000): 154–60.

Zhan, S., and S. C. Ho. "Meta-Analysis of the Effects of Soy Protein Containing Isoflavones on the Lipid Profile." *American Journal of Clinical Nutrition* 81, no. 2 (February 2005): 397–408.

Chapter 6: Healing Herbs and Spices

Aggarwal, B. B., and S. Shishodia. "Suppression of the Nuclear Factor-κ B Activation Pathway by Spice-Derived Phytochemicals: Reasoning for Seasoning." *Annals of the New York Academy of Science* 1030 (December 2004): 434–41.

Ali, B. H., and G. Blunden. "Pharmacological and Toxicological Properties of *Nigella Sativa*." *Phytotherapy Research* 17, no. 4 (April 2003): 299–305.

al-Sereiti, M. R., K. M. Abu-Amer, and P. Sen. "Pharmacology of Rosemary (*Rosmarinus Officinalis Linn.*) and Its Therapeutic Potentials." *Indian Journal of Experimental Biology* 37, no. 2 (February 1999): 124–30.

American Spice Trade Association.

Anderson, R. A., C. L. Broadhurst, M. M. Polansky, W. F. Schmidt, A. Khan, V. P. Flanagan, N. W. Schoene, and D. J. Graves. "Isolation and Characterization of Polyphenol Type-A Polymers from Cinnamon with Insulin-Like Biological Activity." *Journal of Agriculture and Food Chemistry* 52, no. 1 (January 14, 2004): 65–70.

Arcila-Lozano, C. C., G. Loarca-Pina, S. Lecona-Uribe, and E. Gonzalez de Mejia. "Oregano: Properties, Composition and Biological Activity." *Archives of Latinoamerican Nutrition* 54, no. 1 (March 2004): 100–111.

Bordia, A., S. K. Verma, and K. C. Srivastava. "Effect of Ginger (*Zingiber Officinale Rosc.*) and Fenugreek (*Trigonella Foenumgraecum L.*) on Blood Lipids, Blood Sugar and Platelet Aggregation in Patients with Coronary Artery Disease." *Prostaglandins, Leukotrienes, and Essential Fatty Acids* 56, no. 5 (May 1997): 379–84.

Broadhurst, C. L., M. M. Polansky, and R. A. Anderson. "Insulin-Like Biological Activity of Culinary and Medicinal Plant Aqueous Extracts in Vitro." *Journal of Agriculture and Food Chemistry* 48, no. 3 (March 2000): 849–52.

Choi, E. M., and J. K. Hwang. "Antiinflammatory, Analgesic and Antioxidant Activities of the Fruit of *Foeniculum Vulgare*." *Fitoterapia* 75, no. 6 (September 2004): 557–65.

Cook, N. C., and S. Samman. "Flavonoids—Chemistry, Metabolism, Cardioprotective Effects, and Dietary Sources." *Journal of Nutritional Biochemistry* 7 (1996): 66–76.

Dhandapani, S., V. R. Subramanian, S. Rajagopal, and N. Namasivayam. "Hypolipidemic Effect of *Cuminum Cyminum L.* on Alloxan-Induced Diabetic Rats." *Pharmacology Research* 46, no. 3 (September 2002): 251–55.

Elson, C. E. "Suppression of Mevalonate Pathway Activities by Dietary Isoprenoids: Protective Roles in Cancer and Cardiovascular Disease." *Journal of Nutrition* 125 (1995): 1666S–1672S.

Fuhrman, B., M. Rosenblat, T. Hayek, R. Coleman, and M. Aviram. "Ginger Extract Consumption Reduces Plasma Cholesterol, Inhibits LDL Oxidation and Attenuates Development of Atherosclerosis in Atherosclerotic, Apolipoprotein E-Deficient Mice." *Journal of Nutrition* 130, no. 5 (May 2000): 1124–31.

Guh, J. H., F. N. Ko, T. T. Jong, and C. M. Teng. "Antiplatelet Effect of Gingerol Isolated from *Zingiber Officinale*." *Journal of Pharmacy and Pharmacology* 47, no. 4 (April 1995): 329–32.

Lal, A. A., T. Kumar, P. B. Murthy, and K. S. Pillai. "Hypolipidemic Effect of *Coriandrum Sativum L.* in Triton-Induced Hyperlipidemic Rats." *Indian Journal of Experimental Biology* 42, no. 9 (September 2004): 909–12.

Manach, C., F. Regerat, O. Texier, et al. "Bioavailability, Metabolism and Physiological Impact of 4-Oxo-Flavonoids." *Nutritional Research* 16 (1996): 517–44.

McCarty, M. F. "Nutraceutical Resources for Diabetes Prevention— an Update." *Med Hypotheses* 64, no. 1 (2005): 151–58.

Nakatani, N. "Chemistry of Antioxidants from Labiatae Herbs." In *Food Phytochemicals for Cancer Prevention II. Teas Spices and Herbs,* eds. M. T. Huang, T. Osawa, C. T. Ho, and R. T. Rosen. Washington, D.C.: American Chemical Society, 1994, 144–53.

Ochiai, T., S. Ohno, S. Soeda, H. Tanaka, Y. Shoyama, and H. Shimeno. "Crocin Prevents the Death of Rat Pheochromyctoma (PC-12) Cells by Its Antioxidant Effects Stronger than Those of Alpha-Tocopherol." *Neuroscience Letters* 362, no. 1 (May 13, 2004): 61–64.

Pearce, B. C., R. A. Parker, M. E. Deason, A. A. Qureshi, and J. J. Wright. "Hypocholesterolemic Activity of Synthetic and Natural Tocotrienols." *Journal of Medical Chemistry* 35 (1992): 3595–606.

Sacchetti, G., A. Medici, S. Maietti, M. Radice, M. Muzzoli, S. Manfredini, E. Braccioli, and R. Bruni. "Composition and Functional Properties of the Essential Oil of Amazonian Basil, *Ocimum Micranthum Willd., Labiatae* in Comparison with Commercial Essential Oils." *Journal of Agriculture and Food Chemistry* 52, no. 11 (June 2, 2004): 3486–91.

USDA-ARS-NGRL. "Phytochemical Database." Beltsville, Maryland: Beltsville Agricultural Research Center.

Verma, S. K., and A. Bordia. "Antioxidant Property of Saffron in Man." *Indian Journal of Medical Science* 52, no. 5 (May 1998): 205–7.

Yazdanparast, R., and M. Alavi. "Antihyperlipidaemic and Antihypercholesterolaemic Effects of *Anethum Graveolens* Leaves After the Removal of Furocoumarins." *Cytobios* 105, no. 410 (2001): 185–91.

Index